D1645836

INTUITIVE WELLNESS

30130 148394538

INTUITIVE WELLNESS

Using Your Body's Inner Wisdom to Heal

Laura Alden Kamm

SIMON &
SCHUSTER

London · New York · Sydney · Toronto

A CBS COMPANY

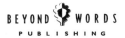

BEYOND WORDS
PUBLISHING

ESSEX COUNTY
COUNCIL LIBRARY

First published in Great Britain by Simon & Schuster UK Ltd, 2007
A CBS COMPANY

Originally published in the US in 2006 by Atria Books/Beyond Words,
an imprint of Simon & Schuster, Inc.

Copyright © 2006 by Laura Alden Kamm
Portions of the introduction appeared in *Hot Chocolate for the Mystical Soul* by
Arielle Ford (Plume Books, 1998).

This book is copyright under the Berne Convention.
No reproduction without permission.
All rights reserved.

The right of Laura Alden Kamm to be identified as author of this work
has been asserted by her in accordance with sections 77 and 78
of the Copyright, Designs and Patents Act, 1988.

1 3 5 7 9 10 8 6 4 2

Simon & Schuster UK Ltd
Africa House
64-78 Kingsway
London WC2B 6AH

www.simonsays.co.uk

Simon & Schuster Australia
Sydney

A CIP catalogue record for this book is available from the British Library

ISBN 13: 978-1-84737-045-7

Printed and bound in Great Britain by
CPI Bath Press

Dedication

With love and gratitude to my parents . . .

Rev. Dr Roland Travers Kamm and Mary Alden Kamm

You taught me to discover the extraordinary in the everyday;
to be of service; to love unconditionally;
and to always seek new horizons.

CONTENTS

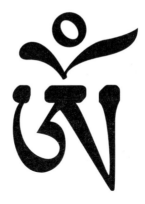

Preface

Pictured above is the Tibetan Buddhist symbol for *om*, the universal harmonic of God. Notice that directly below the circle are two lines that resemble a bird's wings. This symbol, with its suggestion of wings, expresses my intention for this book. Aviation engineers know the theoretical mechanics of flight and can help a person wishing to understand flight, but their experience is in the realm of theory. If you wanted to learn how to fly, you would prefer that a pilot teach you, and your best teacher would be someone who knew both theory and its application. Like other great philosophies, Buddhism teaches that in order for a person to achieve enlightenment, or God consciousness, he or she needs to apply both innate wisdom and the wisdom that has been learned from life and teachers. This book, too, is meant to offer ideas and principles and their practical application—so you yourself can learn how to fly.

All along my life's path, I have been drawn into body experience first and later stumbled upon the literature to back up or validate my experience. This is perhaps the path of an empathic person. To learn something, we've got to get it into the body first. This way of experiencing life gives greater depth of understanding to our journey. Luckily, we are all empathic to varying degrees, and therefore this idea applies to all of us. In order for us to learn something, really learn and embrace it, we have to direct it into our bodies.

As a child I knew that all paths lead to the same door, and that there are just different ways to knock. My spiritual experiences in childhood demonstrated this to me very clearly. As I grew into an adult, a life-threatening illness brought forth many physical, mental, and spiritual challenges and experiences. Afterward, literature from ancient religions and philosophies helped me to be at peace with these soulful experiences and encounters.

Look again at the wings of the symbol for *om*. Just as a bird or butterfly needs two wings to fly to its destination, you also need two wings as you fly through your life toward enlightenment. One wing, the left wing, is your innate wisdom and the wisdom you gain from knowledge and understanding of the world in and around you as you experience it. It is your feminine nature, the divine mother who carries the consciousness of intuition. Your intuition and its further development will bring you greater knowledge of self and deeper levels of understanding, from which your wisdom will develop and grow.

The other wing, the right wing, is the masculine, the divine father, the consciousness through which action is applied. It is the wing of method.

My prayer is that this book will provide you with a sampling of both wisdom and method, which simply need to be awakened and recognized as already within you. As you read and work with what resonates for you in this book, I am confident that your own wings of wisdom and method will emerge, helping you fly home to your source with greater harmony and peace.

Acknowledgments

Life is not a solo act, although at times, we'd like to think otherwise. We need others to support, guide, and encourage us along the way. To that end, my gratitude goes to Cynthia Black and Richard Cohn at Beyond Words Publishing for believing in my work and its message. The opportunity to walk this part of the journey with you is a joy. To the "village" at Beyond Words Publishing who raised this book, my enormous appreciation goes to all. To the Managing Editor, Henry Covi; you made navigating the "big league" publishing industry seamless. To Rachel Berry, Marie Hix, and Carol Sibley, and special thanks to Julie Steigerwaldt for her editing contributions; many thanks to all of you for your long hours and dedication to this work. Sincere thanks goes to the staff at Simon & Schuster for their guidance and long-reaching arm.

To my literary agent Lynn Franklin: Lynn, thank you for standing with me through the years. I genuinely rely on your expertise and wisdom. I would also like to express my gratitude to Amy Armstrong, Sherry Butler, and Vivian Glyck. I am so grateful for your friendships, insight, and support; you have helped me beyond measure

To Mike Ashby: Thank you for your editing contribution. You masterfully sculpted this work so it could be presented to a larger audience. I could not have done this foundational work without you. Thank you! I also wish to offer my appreciation to Corey Deitz, John Kamm, and E. J. Sexton for their generous contributions of time and support in the realm of the Internet.

I would also like to acknowledge Dr. Gladys Taylor McGarey, "the mother of holistic medicine," for her contribution to the original manuscript. Dr. Gladys, you inspire so many and our world is a better, healthier place because of you.

My love and appreciation goes to Sandra Janzen for being a person of destiny in the relay of life. You were the hand-off person, gifting me with a little book you thought I'd enjoy. Your act of kindness delivered what was "next" in my life and opened new horizons.

Finally, to those who stand closest to me: I want to thank my parents Mary and Rollie, my bother and sisters, John, Christine, and Kate; and my children Alicia and Christopher. Thank you for the love, joy, and laughter you bring to my life. To Geoffrey Morris; your love and encouragement to "stay on the path" has been invaluable. As Joseph Campbell said, "The privilege of a lifetime is to be yourself." I'm grateful our family lives this way.

My heartfelt appreciation goes to my clients and students; it is for you that I share this message. I am honored to be a part of your lives. You are the true pioneers of healing.

May you be happy
May you be healthy
May you be free

Introduction

The body never lies. It always knows the truth of any situation, because it is through the body that our soul speaks to us. The body is the temple of the soul.

My initiation into this profound understanding and into becoming a healer and medical intuitive—someone with the capability to determine disorders and diseases through intuiting and "seeing" energy—came wrapped in mind-searing pain and a life-threatening illness. Throughout this ordeal, a faint, long-forgotten voice revealed a wisdom hidden deep within that guided me through a miraculous recovery. My soul was crying out to me from the heart of my shattered temple.

In 1982, at twenty-six years old, I suffered through a painful and perplexing illness. Seven months earlier, I asked my doctor to examine a cyst located at the back of my head, something that had been there since birth. He assured me that it could easily be removed in his office and did so at that time. But we did not know that it was a rare kind of cyst. Only much later, after my illness had taken its course, did we learn that the cyst had formed while I was in my mother's womb and was in fact the beginning of another child—my twin. Unfortunately, my twin didn't form beyond a few cells. But those cells lodged in my head while I was developing, creating the cyst.

When my illness began, I awoke with a severe headache and vomiting. My doctor found no connection to the cyst that had been removed. Instead, the diagnosis was flu and a sinus infection, and he sent me home with medication and the usual instructions to drink lots of liquid and get plenty of rest. But with every passing day, my symptoms worsened. In five days I lost seventeen pounds from my relentless retching. A voice inside my head kept warning me that this wasn't the flu, that something was terribly wrong.

Gradually, as the days passed and my illness progressed, I realized the wisdom of this inner voice. It was a source of strength that had once guided me when I was very young, but had since receded from my consciousness. For years, I had been too busy preoccupied with life—living out my role as mother, wife, and college student—to hear it. These demands had cut me off from my deeper self, my fundamental being, and my spiritual core, so much so that I had even forgotten the concept and was no longer tethered to my own truth and inner wisdom. As a result, the deepest and truest aspects of myself had been lying dormant for years. Now my soul was unearthing my long-buried wisdom, crying out through my illness.

Because I had lost so much body fluid from the constant vomiting, I checked myself into the hospital about a week after my illness set in. It was obvious to me that I had crossed a threshold. Diagnostic tests were run to pin down the cause of my mysterious illness. Then the pain in my head became unbearable, and my eyes started to protrude. My frustrated doctors frantically ordered test after test.

Lying in my hospital bed, I tried to listen more closely to my inner voice. Though I now knew there was something vital about its inner presence and its connection to my illness, I was frustrated because, although it murmured some form of internal distress signal from my soul, it offered no precise information about what was really happening. In the hopes of fine-tuning my inner voice's message, I would squirm around, moving my legs up and down. I would try to swing one of them over the bed railing, but was too weak to move it all the way over. Sometimes I would let it hang off the bed until the nurse came back to my room and put it back. She would then pack pillows around me but there was no way my painful body could find comfort. My attempts to move around were futile, and I felt greater and greater unease as the pain in my head became thunderous and out of control.

I could feel the life-force energy that had filled and supported my body drying up. I knew I was facing death. As I clung to life, my heart reached out to hold onto my husband, parents, brother and sisters, friends, and my two beautiful young children, Alicia and Christopher. I wanted to watch my children grow up. I wanted them to remember their mother, and how much I loved them. I wanted to share with them the things I had been taught and shown as a child, which had meant so much to me. I was afraid I would only be remembered through some worn photographs, hardly capable of expressing my face, my actions, and my love for them. My body was soaked in panic as I lay alone and powerless.

Each time I gazed at myself in the bathroom mirror, waves of horror swept over me. Who belonged to this face? My skin had taken on a foreign color and texture, a sallow greenish-gray, and my eyes bulged ghoulishly from their sockets. The me I knew was disappearing, being replaced by someone who was beyond sickly. Where was I going, and why was I leaving?

On the morning of the eleventh day of my illness, I lay surrounded by my loving family and worried doctors. All of them sensed my impending death. As I observed the bewildered faces around me, I sensed that something inside me was changing. My inner voice was giving me clearer direction. And, as my inner knowing burgeoned forth with fresh awareness, I sensed a new journey unfolding. To my surprise, I no longer shared the concern of those gathered around me.

My awareness of physical reality, an imprisoning reality that I had constructed within the shallow limits of my five senses, was starting to fade. My spirit was beginning preparations for its transcendence. Muted impressions of peace began to weave through my body, and I knew that these sensations of tranquility were indications of what was to come. I began to realize that everything that was happening to me imbued with an exalted purpose and was orchestrated by some universal force.

Later that afternoon, when my family had left to let me rest, I was finally alone with this new awareness. The chronic sensations of foreboding were gone, and the pain, which had become a part of me, had transmuted itself ever so gently. My mind and sensations were passing through a gateway to a different dimension, a new level of consciousness.

Without warning or provocation, I began to witness with my physical eyes what I could only describe as my soul lifting up and floating away. Watching intently, I saw and felt the vigor of my soul lighten as it floated upward, forming itself into a beautiful, pale, bluish-white fog hovering four to six inches above my stomach and lower abdomen. All at once, this part of my body, from which my energy or soul had left, changed color to a heavy, sodden gray. I watched as the same process was repeated with sections of my legs and arms. It finally moved through the trunk of my body, engulfing me in a thick, heavy feeling.

I became aware of a system that consisted of multidimensional layers of my being, and I found myself attempting to identify the particulars within each layer. But they were only slightly perceptible. Interpreting them was difficult, as I had no framework or reference point for such an experience. Still, my curiosity pressed forward, continuing to observe and feel into what seemed to be four or five magical layers.

It was as if someone had turned on a movie inside my head. My mind's eye, or inner vision, became extraordinarily lucid, and I was seeing in a strange and seemingly magical way. I could see the spaces between the walls of my physical body. Whether my eyes were open or closed, I could see the bones, the muscles, and the blood. While I continued to observe my soul pulling itself away from my physical being like taffy, my new inner vision took me into different levels of consciousness. At times I actually felt that I had some control over the process. Looking at the outside of my body, I could see energy moving in and around me. Turning my attention back inside my body, I was able to see into the bones and tissues of my legs and study the myriad colorful energies dancing all about.

I could visually telescope down into the empty spaces and watch with even greater clarity as my soul left what appeared to be the molecules and atoms that constructed my body. By some mysterious force, I saw deep within the infinitesimal parts of my body and observed the miraculous separation of spirit and matter.

Although I didn't fully understand what was happening, I did realize several things. I instinctively knew that my role was to be an observer, to let things happen, and to pay attention: I was not to have much control over this vision. Still, I had no clue as to the origin of this projector-like way of seeing. Everything was transpiring so quickly.

It seemed as though my body's energy was intertwining with something distant and unnamed. The light of my soul was also changing and I could feel its effervescent energy leaving. Ironically, as this bubbling essence lifted away, my heart felt lighter. I felt stronger, or perhaps it was my consciousness that felt stronger, as the sensation of my body continued to drift into a seemingly detached, heavy-feeling place of "nonexistence."

Before this illness, I had been unaware of the river of energy that flowed inside me. Now I was conscious that this life force was beginning its unconstrained journey to its true home. An ancient, innate wisdom flowed little by little through my consciousness. Freedom and serenity suddenly swept through me and I knew who I was, where I had come from, and what my purpose for being was. More importantly, I was no longer afraid. Along with this awareness came its companion: peace.

Relief engulfed me like torrential floodwaters overflowing their once-restrictive gates. I felt drenched with serenity; nothing earthly mattered. My soul's journey was simply moving to another dimension. Soon I would become once again a more aware and divine being of energy. I was returning to the place where God and I were one.

Bliss completely erased all prior concerns regarding my earthly existence. Now I knew I would always be connected to my family and friends. Because of our spiritual bond, they would never forget me. Thoughts, feelings, and memories would always keep us linked. We would see each other again. So often we think of birth as creation and death as an end. But the glorious peace I was experiencing within the multi-sensory levels of my being was by no means an end—it was creation ablaze! A lightness and interconnectedness with all souls filled me. I was dying and at the same time being set free.

A whirling sound drifted slowly into my ears and head, rising and falling melodiously. The tone encircled me with peculiar familiarity that felt comforting. Thoughts continually streamed through my mind, reassuring me that it was no longer necessary to suffer.

But my soul did not completely leave my body that afternoon. Instead I fell into a deep sleep.

Evening arrived, along with visitors. As they sat talking on the edge of my bed, their words passed over me. I was awake, but my mind was probing deep within, trying to remember everything I had experienced that afternoon. Had I been dreaming? My logical, rational mind tried to discount what had happened but my heart's wisdom proclaimed the truth: This was a sacred rite of passage. My soul's exodus had indeed begun that afternoon.

Late that night, hearing my cries for help, nurses raced into my room. I had gotten out of bed, gone into the bathroom, and come out screaming, "I can't see! I'm blind!" My eyes were protruding from their sockets to a degree the nurses had never seen. Doctors were summoned and my family called. An immediate transfer by ambulance to another hospital twenty-five miles away was ordered.

I have no memory of yelling for the nurses or of telling them I was blind. Nor do I remember being loaded into the ambulance. But I do remember floating inside a womb of gentle darkness, a place of peace, warmth, and love that was reminiscent of the bliss of the day before. Now this sensation encompassed my whole being. I was surrounded by a warm, dark, gel-like substance that breathed life, yet held within it death—a void.

Then, as if arising from a deep sleep, my consciousness began to shift. A faint vibrating tone arose somewhere around me and grew more pronounced as it came closer. It raised no fear in me because it was familiar. I remembered its velvety feel from the day before. Suddenly I broke free from the restful state, vibrant and full of energy. At first, I didn't recognize that I had no physical body, that it lay forgotten on the gurney. My soul and my consciousness were up in a corner of the ambulance looking down at a pale, grayish woman. I watched detached as the nurse leaned forward, listening for breath and calling out for me to hold on.

I was glad to be free of a body so obviously riddled with the scourge of disease. Hovering in the ambulance, I became aware that not even the ambulance's tangible barriers could hold my spirit. I was actually able to float through the sides of the vehicle and still maintain a clear view of all that was happening.

Total liberation swept over me as I understood that I was returning to the domain of the spirit. At that point, I experienced an acceptance of my most recent past, causing an immediate emotional disconnection from the ashen body lying there. I now knew that this earthly body and existence were only a tiny part of the whole truth. Surrounded by a feeling of freedom and heading to my place of origin, I soared onward into a place commonly known as "the tunnel."

Though I was flying upward at unparalleled speeds, my journey through the tunnel, which radiated striations of white, soft pink, green, and blue light, was not the least bit dizzying to my senses. Like a hurtling comet, I went through the earthly boundaries. The whirling sound was the same I had heard the day before. Having it wrap around me again felt penetrating and reassuring. There was no fear. In fact, I embraced this place.

I realized that I had a new body, similar to the one I had left behind but better balanced, more buoyant, and full of energy. Information filled my mind and heart, and I realized that this body was the essence that had made up the body I had on earth. This was the life force I had watched disengage from my physical body during the afternoon in the hospital. Made of light, love, and a powerful pulsating energy, I could hardly believe I felt so fabulous and so full of love for myself and my surroundings.

Approaching the end of the tunnel, I was catapulted out with a force so powerful that it propelled me into the light. My arms and legs were flailing. In a feeble human attempt to keep from falling, I reached to grab the emptiness. Awkward and off balance, I realized I had not fully let go of my humanness. As I look back I think how ridiculous it was to be flailing around, clutching for something to hold onto. I was dead. My spirit was fully alive in its most natural state. Yet my consciousness was still embedded with human-constructed realities and attempting to control things the old way. I had not fully let go.

Colliding with the full force of this powerful light, I felt like my breath had been taken away, as if I had taken the summer's first plunge into a glacial lake. My surge of panic was gone, and I drifted into the love-filled light. I gasped with wonderment and childlike exhilaration as I was surrounded by the Light of God, love, and universal intelligence, which all seemed to be the same thing. I received answers to a lifetime of questions. Strangely, memories of being here before came soaring back in resounding bursts of energy, returning to their proper place within the very fiber of my soul. This was my place of origin. I was home.

I began to feel the presence of angels. The misty veil lifted, and around me stood magnificent beings. Somehow I knew they had been waiting for me, and their warmth embraced me. Communication was telepathic, from heart to heart and smile to smile. No words were spoken aloud. There was no judgment. As their welcoming words rang in my heart, I felt reassured. I understood every word as they guided me back to a full state of awareness, helping me remember who I was and who they were. We communed like this for what seemed to be a long time.

Then I became aware that I was in another place, surrounded by volumes and volumes of huge books. Some of the books were opened for me, and on the pages were scenes from my life playing out like a movie. I vividly recall one scene from when I was five or six. It was a beautiful spring day and my best friend and I were doing our usual investigation of the neighborhood. I thought it would be a great idea for us to find a baby robin's egg, hatch it, and raise it ourselves. I had always wanted to have a robin for a pet. It wasn't long before we found a nest cradled in a neighbor's ladder, which hung on the side of the garage.

The taller of the two, I had the job of reaching into the tightly woven nest to grab an egg. In our search for adventure, we had forgotten about the mother robin. Suddenly she came darting toward my hand and head, chirping frantically and flapping her wings. My friend and I ducked and dodged the parental squawks and, somehow, I managed to hang onto the egg.

We dashed toward my friend's backyard where, seated at a picnic table, we gently chipped and peeled away the protective layers of the egg, birthing the baby bird ourselves. But our excitement quickly turned to dread, as the tiny creature looked nothing like the baby robin we were expecting. It was feeble and featherless, and soon it was dead. We sat regarding our deed in horror-filled silence.

Now, in the presence of angels, remorse welled up in me. I could feel not only my own pain and sorrow, but my friend's as well. And even more, I felt and absorbed the mother robin's panic and sorrow as she searched for her unborn baby. But the worst sensation was that of the unborn baby robin, as I could feel the energy that was once inside that tiny, helpless creature. I felt an overwhelming sense of loss for all. I was devastated beyond anything I might have felt on earth. The heaviness of this burden gave me a deep awareness of the interconnectedness of all things.

Then, without warning, a gargantuan being came up behind me. The male-feeling energy loomed thirty to forty feet high. I had no need to turn to see it. I could feel its overwhelmingly loving presence, which made me feel like a child. This being conveyed the understanding that I would be most welcome to stay here, but I still had some tasks to accomplish, and it would be most beneficial for my soul's growth and evolution to return to my life and attend to these matters. Images of my children's faces and my family flashed through my mind, and I knew what my heart and soul had decided.

"Do you know where you are? Do you know your name? Do you know who the president is?"

This wasn't a radiant being talking to me; it was the nurse in the neuro-ICU unit at the hospital. I was awakening from a coma. They were explaining to me what had happened. It was so hard to return to earthly reality and listen.

The hospital tests had finally discovered abscesses in the right occipital lobe of my brain, residual complications from the cyst that had been removed seven months earlier. On top of that I had a severe case of spinal meningitis, and the resulting increase in fluid had caused my eyes to protrude from their sockets as the liquid tried to find some point of release. Because the abscessed material had woven itself through my brain, intricate and risky surgery was necessary.

Within only a few months after the surgery, I had physically recovered from the ordeal and my strength slowly returned. Fortunately, I had regained all but a portion of my eyesight. But I was still blind in the left visual field of both eyes, which created challenges. I wasn't able to drive, I was dependent on others to help with everyday errands, and I was bruised all over the left side of my body from bumping into things.

I was relieved to be through with the ordeal, but then, eight months after the surgery, I began to see strange things. I was sure that the illness was returning. Perhaps my doctor had not removed all the abscessed material. Bands and circles of colors seemed to surround everything. At first, I started to see colors around birds and plants, but soon I was seeing colors around people. I kept this development to myself. I was convinced that everyone would think I was crazy, primarily because I believed it myself.

Finally I confessed this development to my doctor, who assured me I was fine and matter-of-factly informed me that I was seeing energy fields. I believed him but was also hesitant. The last time I had seen this type of energy I was sixteen. Then, when I shared the experience, those in authority other than my parents told me that what I had seen and felt didn't exist. So it was the young girl in me who resisted the doctor's information. How could energy exist now when I had been told that it didn't exist then?

Years passed and I kept my near-death experience to myself. How could I describe something so foreign anyway? But I felt very alone with it. I did find out that my sister and a close friend both "saw" me on the day of my near-death experience. The visitations happened just minutes apart, despite the fact that they lived in different states. Apparently, I had come to say good-bye. This was the only validation of all I had experienced and it helped me to believe that what I remembered was true.

My work as a medical intuitive began quite accidentally shortly thereafter. Early one day, my husband accidentally slammed the trunk lid of the car on his hand. I cupped his hand in mine, and as I held it my hands suddenly became very hot. Then the telescoping vision, the same kind of detailed vision I had experienced during my illness and had not seen since, reappeared. I found myself staring at a vivid, hot red and yellow core that represented the pain he was experiencing deep within his hand. And I heard and sensed the screams of pain from each of the affected cells.

Then everything clicked. A cosmic wheel had finally found its notch, allowing it to turn unencumbered and without struggle. I now knew what was happening with my hands, and my altered state of vision seemed normal. Stability and calm came over me. After a few minutes, I let go of his hands and the visions and sensations let go as well.

The next morning, the children and I had just finished breakfast when my husband came downstairs waving his hand, exclaiming, "I don't know what you did to my hand yesterday, but it doesn't hurt any-more." I wasn't sure either, but I knew I wanted to learn more.

Fortunately, I met a woman who was to put my experiences into perspective and allow me to move forward with greater understanding. Sharon owned a business next door to mine. We first met when I went into her store. On the wall was a calendar with a picture of a large tree in a forest. Tiny lights like fairy lights emanated from a large hollow at the base of the tree. Turning toward Sharon, I said, "I believe in that stuff. I see things like that all the time."

As it turned out, so did Sharon, and she also did intuitive readings. We chatted awhile, and then I made an appointment with her for a reading at her house.

Sitting in her home, I listened to Sharon tell me I was a healer, that I could indeed "see," and that I needed to get busy and direct that seeing ability so that I could allow this gift to expand to its fullest extent. My path was finally cleared that day, and I have never looked back.

Since accepting my gift as an intuitive and a healer, I have spent the last twenty years working with thousands of people who want to be healed or who want to learn how to heal themselves and their loved ones. I have studied with Tibetan Rinpoches and Lamas and with Lakota and Yaqui medicine men and women. Before my transforming illness, I had been educated in the field of construction design and technology. However, with the loss of my eyesight I could not see well enough to draw blueprints. Computer-aided drafting techniques were not available at that time, so I turned my academic attention toward the field of applied medical anthropology, the study of cross-cultural healing techniques. Now I am described as a "cartographer of consciousness," a mapmaker of the mind, because of my ability to assist others in mapping their energetic patterns and transforming their deepest fears into positive, inspired, and creative action.

In the intuitive assessments I conduct with clients, I work to discern what is going on within a client's body and its various systems—both physical and energetic. This is where the vision I developed after my near-death experience comes into play. I scan a client's body and see subtle biochemical imbalances and microscopic disorders. I sense the speed and direction with which a disease is forming and spreading, even before a CAT scan or MRI can detect it. Additionally, I observe the emotional and behavioral components surrounding the organs, soft tissue, and bones. Along with this, I work with clients to address the emotional and behavioral components of disorders, misalignments, and diseases, as well as the important relationships in their lives. Finally, we work together to address the soul and the issues that are yearning to come forth.

Some people say that I have a gift: the gift of vision and intuition. I believe that my natural intuitive abilities, which I have experienced in varying degrees since childhood, were brought to the forefront of my awareness by my near-death experience. After that, my intuitive and inner seeing abilities took on the qualities of a gift—something suddenly and surprisingly given. However, I know that intuition is a natural part of our humanness. I tell every client that what I can do, they can do for themselves and most likely for others. You truly are your own healer.

Using This Book

Developing your intuition takes practice. To assist you in this, useful, practical, and effective exercises are included in the back of the book. They have proven to be highly valuable to my students and clients, and have played a crucial role in their intuitive training. I urge you to make them a part of your everyday life.

All the exercises in this book are intuitively driven. You have to engage your intuition to reap their benefits. You will strengthen your intuitive skill just by playing around with them and then practicing them in earnest. It is an evolutionary process and you need to be willing to put in some time every day in order to develop your intuition.

At first, the exercises and their application to your life and learning might seem difficult or confusing. But I assure you, they will help you gain a more spiritual and intellectual understanding. They will also give you a greater sense of body awareness; and once it gets into your body, the densest part of yourself, you've got it!

I encourage you to get the mechanics of each exercise down, and then practice it whenever you are called to by your body's wisdom. You—your body, mind, and spirit—want wellness and healing. Wellness requires regular maintenance because both your internal and external environments are constantly changing, as all things do. So return to the exercises that resonate with you as often as you can.

You may find that the exercises will "stir your pot," revealing things that have been held in your emotional being that might be uncomfortable to look at. Rest assured, however, that I have encountered no instances in my years of experience in which people found out more about themselves than they could handle. Looking at the depth and breadth of who and where you currently are, as well as being willing to expand yourself even further, is what spiritual work is all about. You would not be reading this book or doing this work if you were not prepared for the adventures that will be brought forth from your soul into your life.

Journaling is another important aspect of your spiritual development. Keep a notebook handy as you read this book to jot down issues that come up for you. Writing down your experience is especially valuable when it comes to the exercises. You will be working through what I call "energy mapping," a process by which you uncover submerged patterns of energy, emotions, thought forms, and behaviors. This involves writing down your experience as though you were simply the observer, thereby reporting objectively. As you work with this exercise over a period of time, patterns of the way your energy flows will begin to emerge. You will discover the "bones" of who you are energetically; you will perceive the energetic structure by which you create and hold onto the thought forms that sustain your reality. This mapping will give you information about the most effective way you can utilize your life-force energy. The skill of mapping also brings forward your ability to intuitively sense specific qualities and both the large and microscopic aspects of that which you are intuiting.

As you read through this book and do its activities, you will see beyond the first-blush meanings of the words to the concepts, energies, and essences that lie behind them. You will discover the universal energy that brings all things into being and through which your growth and evolution are assured. The shift will happen for you as it has for my tens of thousands of clients and students. Your awareness of life will deepen, and your intuitive, mental, and physical well-being will unfurl. With the benefit of your dedication and practice, your sense of self and of the eternity of your being will sharpen and bring you great joy.

1
Discovering Your Soul's Voice

We are experiencing an ever-widening global culture. This stage of our evolution asks us to embrace a state of mind that opens new levels of consciousness and promises balance and healing. The call comes to us in many forms. As a medical intuitive, I see many people in whom the subtle messages of their bodies in the form of aches, pains, or disease urge them to become more aware of their interconnectedness to all things—energetically, physically, spiritually, and mentally. Beyond the healing of our bodies, there is also a cry for healing, and for the state of equanimity that it brings, within the larger cultural and global community. We have not been taking care of ourselves and our communities, and to remedy that, we need to step forward into a new way of living, a new way of being well. It is time to participate in the changes that are part of the natural evolutionary process of consciousness that is now quietly ascending, as it has before in various global cultures throughout time.

I was once on an airplane returning from Southeast Asia. As far as I could tell, I was the only white woman on the huge Boeing 747. I sat in the middle of the plane with my eyes closed, feeling like the only stranger in a crowd. But then someone sneezed, and it sounded just like one of my sneezes. We are all inherently the same, I thought; we come from the same cosmic force. Outward differences and illusions of separateness keep us from embracing our oneness and chain our perceptions to the false dualism of self and other.

Consciousness is expanding rapidly in people. Synchronistic events, which are indications of a greater awareness of the interconnectedness of life, are becoming more widespread. People who have pursued a spiritual path for a long time are reaching even greater dimensions of consciousness. We can all be of assistance to others along the journey of our souls' growth.

Encountering the crossroads along the pathway of this evolutionary process of consciousness sometimes creates disquiet. The journey can indeed be tumultuous. Yet it is time to shift again and awaken to multidimensional streams of thought and reality. The old paradigm, representing a disconnected and less compassionate way of living, is crumbling. A timeless shifting of consciousness is occurring within and around us. It is up to us to be aware, attentive, and willing to meet this destined shift.

Consciousness is directly related to illness, misalignment, and disease. It has become clear from my experience as a medical intuitive that our way of living—our spiritual, mental, and physical habits—dictates our state of being. Furthermore, our states of awareness are affected by the condition of our being. For instance, it is difficult to be spiritually awake while suffering from addictive habits. Our perceptions and beliefs, our emotions and thoughts about our health and wellness, reside in those states of consciousness.

When we come from a place of deep awareness and understanding regarding our wellness, we bring about change not only within ourselves but also within the larger community. If these words resonate with you, perhaps it is time to explore your own nature and embrace the eternal existence of the unified self and of your communal destiny. It may be time to consider changing how you care for your body and soul.

Concepts regarding the calling forth of our soulful nature have been illuminated since the beginning of time. Accomplishing this leap will require you to understand deeply what is happening in both the interior and exterior arenas of your personal world. Help will come to you naturally, however, because as you make individual shifts and gain new levels of awareness and consciousness, you will automatically join with like-minded others. The resulting group energy propels all of us to a quantum leap in consciousness.

Evidence of this is all around us. Television and movies reflect these spiritual changes and consequently the way we think and operate in the world. Practices such as yoga and tai chi, which were once hidden as mystical arts, are commonplace. Baby boomers and their kids are assured that they can have a lifestyle that combines organic foods, meditation, and Wall Street. It's not just a marketing phenomenon. Spirituality has always been here, and evolution has brought it out of the dark recesses of the world's monasteries and into our living rooms. We have indeed arrived at a marvelous, albeit precarious, point in the evolution of our consciousness. We are poised at a place where we can learn to heal our world and ourselves by applying our innate wisdom—intuition.

As we watch consciousness shift in and around us, we return quite naturally to certain fundamental questions: Who am I? What is my life's purpose? Where did I come from? Why am I here? This change is organic, contained within a natural and universal set of protocols. When change and the suffering that sometimes comes with it occur, we ultimately turn inward to connect with the energy that is in turn connected to Spirit. We want to become solidly joined with it, not apart from it. We go into the deep recesses of ourselves if for no other reason than to ask questions of who, what, where, and why. We all know what this feels like; we have all asked the questions, often with heartfelt anguish. You wonder why you have a disease, why someone you love has died, why it hurts so much trying to fit in. And the answer may never come. We learn that life is messy and hard. We also yearn for those moments of peace, pleasure, and joy.

Our brains are squeezed with confused thoughts. Our body's biochemistry shifts, leading ultimately to reactive emotions and physical ailments. Contending with these intimate enemies is probably tougher than confronting any external adversary. But once you decide to become your own healer, the light will begin to shine and healing will take place. Your life and consciousness will change as you engage in the power of your intuition, your soul's voice. Through your inner work, your questions will be answered. And any part of your voice that has been silenced, and any aspect of your life that has been paralyzed, will be free.

The Proper Care and Feeding of Your Soul

Your spirit animates your body and mind, expressing itself through your personality. The process of fully realizing this spiritual connection is gradual and cannot be forced. To properly care for and feed your soul, which is the basis of your being's wellness, it is necessary to realize that you are a soul, an essence of pure mind and heart manifesting a specific vibration, whose destiny is, at some point in boundless time, to be filled with the pure light of consciousness, the light of God. As such, you are in fact already whole and perfect in God's eyes, no matter what occurs in your life or your physical body. You undertake this journey, which leads you through the process of self-discovery (realization of your connection to God) and onward into self-mastery (actualization of the God within you).

So, although you are already whole and a part of you is perfectly enlightened, all the things you have experienced in your life have been opportunities for you to grow. You might be able to see instances in your past of your soul's desire to help you evolve. Your soul has been escorting you through the vast banquet of your life experiences, using your emotions to give those events form and place them firmly in the anatomy of your spirit, mind, and body. It is important to become aware of this process and manage it consciously through choice and free will—not willfulness—to bring about the alignment and liberation of your soul. By participating in this process, you will release your soul, mind, and body from pain, ignorance, and suffering.

Nurturing your awareness and listening within as deeply as you can will bring you guidance. Finally, fixing a place of even-mindedness within your emotional being will foster inner knowing and peace.

Your Invitation to a New Way of Living

In the past, when teaching intuitive development and energy medicine, I made it a practice never to tell students what would occur in their lives when they did their homework—some of which you will find as exercises in the back of this book. I mentioned possibilities, but did not necessarily give actual examples of change other students had experienced. One night, however, a student changed my mind about this policy. It was the third of four (biweekly) classes, and the students were beginning their fifth week of exercises. As always, I held a check-in time at the beginning of class to see how everyone was doing.

Hannah raised her hand and laughingly said to me, "How come you didn't tell us that this class would change our lives?" I explained that after committing to this type of work, I had always seen profound changes in people and their lives. I didn't mention anything, I continued, because I didn't want to program the students; I wanted everyone to be completely open to his or her own particular experience without any expectations or influence from others' experiences. Hannah then told me that she was okay with the fact that her life had changed so dramatically since she had started taking the course and doing the exercises, but she wished that I had told her just how much it was about to change. She related that she had recently spent five days with her best friend of the last twelve years, and that during their time together she realized that she no longer had anything in common with this woman. She was surprised by her discovery of how much her class work had caused shifts and changes in her.

Hannah understood more clearly than ever before what served her in her life and what didn't. Through her new dedication to her spiritual practice and her experiences with the class exercises, she had gained a deeper understanding of what she needed in her life. Her soul had said "Hello!" It had been a powerful experience for her. She owned who she was and what she wanted to become, realizing that appeasement would no longer be a part of her life; no longer would she stay in a relationship—any relationship—that didn't move her toward growth.

Occasionally during our healing process we step away from active participation in healing and simply let things simmer inside. This allows the work to percolate, and sometimes events occur that bring about the next cycle of our life and our healing. James's story demonstrates this perfectly. In the two years I had been working with him, I felt privileged to assist him in resolving some deep early childhood scars and wounds; however, he continued to assert control over the things and people around him in order to feel safe. His heart was shut down and his feelings for his spouse waxed and waned. One day as I was working with him, I placed my hand on his chest, and the impact of energy from the buildup of congestion there was so strong that it caused a bruise in a vein in my hand that remained for several days.

The energy around his heart had concretized, and I knew he needed to just sit with the work we had been doing. As a facilitator of healing, I listened to my client's voice. I sensed that his path would soon unfold. A few months later, I got a call from his wife telling me he had been rushed to the hospital with heart problems requiring a stent in one of his arteries. Our work began again.

James is a different man now. The loving, gentle heart he came into this world with has been reborn, and all aspects of his life—physical, emotional, and mental—are healing. It took a life-threatening situation for him to finally understand that being too controlling was unhealthy for him. He realized how much better it would be if people "got it" before facing their own mortality, and he is now an inspiration to others around him.

A Healing Partnership

My intention in the classroom, my office, and in this book is to help others reach an understanding of their souls' existence and, more importantly, discover whatever messages are trapped in their bodies' physical and energetic structures. If I can do this, then I have best served my purpose.

Here is a little lesson I learned from my father while I was visiting my parents years ago. My father often carried his dog, Fritzie, around in his arms like an infant. This intrigued me, and so I teasingly said to him, "Daddy, Fritzie can walk. You know?" My father stopped, nuzzled up against Fritzie's face, and proudly replied, "Yes, Fritzie can walk. But isn't it nice that he doesn't have to?"

I laughed as I understood that his story was telling me what it means to serve others. I know with certainty that we all have the ability to heal ourselves and bring about our own wellness. But there are times when we need a little assistance and guidance from an outside source. And that is my prayer—to be there for someone if they need a little help. A Buddhist prayer runs, in part, "May I be a protector for all who need one. May I be a ship, a boat, a raft for all who wish to cross the water." Serving as a vessel or catalyst to help another person cross the waters of life is a wonderful way of being. All things exist conditionally and therefore appear separate. However, we are all one, so when you help others, you are also helping yourself.

You can indeed do your own healing, or at least be in charge of the healing team you gather around you, but when you need a little help you will find others who will hold you warmly in their arms. It is infinitely rewarding to help others and be helped along your spiritual path.

One day a brilliant young woman named Sally came to me for assistance in correcting her vision. She was studying to be a doctor, and her schedule was hectic. We made some progress in the first session or two, which allowed her to go without her glasses for a short time. Because she had spontaneously experienced clear vision before and after working with me, she was convinced that she should be able to see all the time without her glasses.

Sally came in for another appointment, and I suggested that she needed to address some emotional issues. It was my understanding, as I read the thought forms in her body's tissues and energy field, that there were some deep emotional scars that needed healing in order for her eyesight to maintain its correction. In short, in order to see, Sally needed to truthfully look at things in her life she hadn't been able to face up to that point. She acknowledged that there were some deep-seated emotional issues from childhood, but because of the demands of medical school, she simply didn't want to stir up that emotional pot just yet.

I was sympathetic, but I was direct in my assessment that her healing must take place in the heart (her emotional eyes) as well as in her physical eyes. The results after this particular session were, if not non-existent, less dramatic. I haven't seen Sally since, but always send her healing whenever she appears in my mind's eye. In any case, she will at some point look at these issues, and in so doing become an even greater doctor than she could have imagined.

I share Sally's story to underline that you are your own healer, and as such you need to be willing to heal. Healing occurs on all levels—emotional, physical, mental, spiritual, and others you may not know by name: levels of consciousness that lie somewhere beyond, in a nameless place. In addition, although I often notice people's tendency to give their healing powers away to others, it's important to own your power to heal yourself. All healing is guided by your will and wrapped in your karma and the will of God or Spirit.

Can You Hear the Call to Deeper Awareness?

Life offers us windows of opportunity to grow spiritually. However, we are not always comfortable with or ready for this insight into the profound. One thing to keep in mind is that you can't be aware of something you cannot hear or experience. Its message will be revealed when the time is right. Whatever gift is hidden within the opportunity, it will circle back around into your life; and at some point in time you will open the window and see what lies beyond it.

The following story shares a time in one soul's life when he just couldn't open the window. Those around him did, so all experiences have their purpose in the end.

Neil was a charming man and seemed to have everything going for him in his life. He was a powerful, internationally recognized businessman, with a beautiful wife and two intelligent young boys poised to follow in his footsteps. He had all the conventional trappings of success. He came to see me on the advice of a mutual friend after he was diagnosed with eighteen brain tumors and a spot on one lung. He was scared of dying. In fact, he was determined not to die. It was simply not in his action plan, which he had laid out in a step-by-step format that allowed him to manage both his personal and professional goals and obtain what he desired.

When I scanned his body, I could see that the cancer was extremely aggressive, much like Neil himself when it came to managing his business and life. Neil and his wife told me that he had just had an MRI, so they knew the locations of the cancerous tumors. I also knew the locations of the tumors, but I sensed that there was more to the picture.

With the inner vision that allows me to detect the directional movement of diseases, I could sense and see the particles of the molecular structure that were beginning to form in Neil's body. I discovered that his cancer was rapidly heading down his spinal cord and into his lymphatic system, and would soon manifest in his legs. I worked on him for about an hour, and through the modulation of energy, several painful issues were brought to the surface for him, along with equally deeply buried tears. We scheduled another appointment, and Neil and his wife left my office.

As part of my spiritual practice, after I've seen all my scheduled clients for the day, I go into a meditative state. From that state, I send prayers and do remote work on anyone who has requested it. After my appointment with Neil, I was deeply moved by his strong desire to be cured. I felt, however, that he needed to do some deep healing. He was open to this idea in his first session but couldn't fully see the emotional pain he had held in for years. He believed in the existence of his soul, and he could certainly feel buried emotions well up when we did energy work together. Nonetheless, he had difficulty conceptualizing an integral view of his body, mind, and soul.

Sitting within the silence of myself, I asked for guidance as to how I could be of service to Neil and his family. What I received was a startling vision of an angel holding a clipboard. Although such a vision might seem bizarre, experience has taught me to trust spirit-guided knowledge and phenomena; they often come in ways that are easy to understand. The message in my mind's eye, responding to my question, came quickly and clearly: "No, time is up. Early November." Following this statement, the angel took a pen and put a check mark on the clipboard—by Neil's name, I assumed.

I felt helpless. But, from this vision and my earlier reading of the cancer's aggressiveness, it was clear that Neil's time was up. All I could do, I decided, was support him and his family in whatever way they wanted. Nonetheless, I still held open a space for a miracle to take place. Using the experiences from my own death-like passage, I tried to help Neil with the pain and fear of his disease and what lay ahead for him.

Neil had a strong will, and he fought his cancer to his very last breath. To him, the cancer was a mistake. He never really opened to the invitation for his soul's growth; nor did he read between the lines of his life. He could not grasp that his choices created and determined his life's direction. He just felt that if he kept pushing, things would move out of the way, sooner or later. He was a sensitive man but never dealt with the emotional hurts that were tucked away inside. He died with his consciousness still holding his pain and suffering. He will awaken and achieve his healing, gaining insight into the interconnectedness of life, even if this awakening occurs in the life after his physical one.

But there is good news! You do not necessarily have to get hit over the head with God's velvet hammer; you don't necessarily need to experience extreme illness or the threat of death to answer the invitation of your soul's evolution. The call to deeper levels of awareness, wellness, and personal growth can come in quieter, simpler ways.

While giving a lecture on medical intuition at a bookstore several years ago, for example, I noticed a young woman who sat smiling through the entire program. At the conclusion of my lecture, she raised her hand and announced that she had to tell the story of how she had come to the lecture that evening. Juliet had been out looking for a new apartment when something inside her told her to go into a bookstore and get a cup of coffee. Although she could have stopped for coffee at any number of other places, her soul, through the voice of her intuition, directed her to the bookstore.

Juliet went on to explain that as soon as she entered the store, she heard an announcement about my lecture and the topic I was going to discuss. And what's more, she added, she had recently received several books from a friend on the topic of my presentation. This series of synchronicities led her to a place where her internal questions could be answered. Now we knew why Juliet had sat grinning through the entire program. Her immediate and active response to the call of her intuition shows that we can step into a new awareness without getting hit over the head.

It is totally up to you to choose to listen and respond to your wisdom—or not. Your intuition is a powerful tool that you can sharpen and hone to the point where you can rely on it in the context of your daily life. The decision to open to and trust what you intuitively get is entirely yours. My prayer is that you will take this simple tool that you were born with and work with it, develop it, and commit to its use. Your life will change.

Recommended Exercises

Creating Sacred Space
Introduction to Your Soul

2

Turning On the Power of Your Intuition

Intuition is a skill we all have. It is insight that comes to us without utilizing our mental qualities of reasoning or analysis. Intuition is powerful, but not in the sense of power *over* something or someone; it is a powerful vehicle that allows us to sense and know our connection to God, the planet, other people, and the consciousness of all things. In utilizing our intuitive abilities, we tap into innate universal wisdom, which opens up the dimension of the "nonlocal mind." By nonlocal mind, I mean one that is connected to all moments in time, as well as to all people and all places. A nonlocal mind knows no physical boundaries; it can go anywhere and explore any dimension because it is one with all things in time and space. This oneness can be achieved through practice and honing our intuitive skills; it is what Eastern religions mean when they refer to enlightenment.

The power and use of your intuitive abilities will allow you to expand your consciousness, awareness, inner seeing and hearing abilities, and feeling nature to their ultimate levels. I sometimes refer to "360-degree vision" in this context; it is as if nothing past, present, or future is veiled from you, no matter where you are or what you choose to focus on.

Developing your intuition will necessarily stretch your consciousness; therefore, changes that affect your pathway through life will occur as you proceed. For instance, your conscious mind may open to the truth about a relationship; you may find that it no longer works for you and you need to say good-bye. That is not an easy thing to think about or go through. However, these changes will ultimately be for your highest good. At times you will find yourself at a crossroads. Deciding whether to let go of people, places, and events that have been a part of your world may not be easy to deal with, but if spiritual growth were easy, we'd all be balls of light right now, not struggling or suffering. Nonetheless, as you go through the necessary changes and arrive at new levels of consciousness, you will experience success: Inner peace will grow from trusting your intuitive wisdom; health and balancing your life's activities will be more attainable; and most importantly, you will be living your life in accordance with your inner wisdom. Although developing your intuition will not always be pleasant, rest assured that if you are true to your path, you will find much joy. The difficulties of making certain choices, which seem so daunting, will diminish dramatically as you become clearer about your spiritually based intentions and purpose in life.

As you open each of your intuitive gates, more and more awareness will come to you. Sometimes this awareness will extend beyond your own life to the people and world around you. As a result, people may seek your assistance. This brings up a key aspect of your intuitive development: paying attention to your integrity. Because of the way your intuitive faculties will affect you through the processes of cause and effect, or karma, it is vital that you carefully consider the way you develop and use them. Balance is essential if you decide to use your intuitive skills to help others. Using your intuitive wisdom for self-care and wellness is instrumental in maintaining balance in yourself as you grow intuitively. Is it for personal gain? Or is it not only for your betterment, but also to lead others to greater awareness? The first choice is a burden laden with dissatisfaction and a sense of suffering. The second, a way of service, is filled with rich rewards on all levels. The quality of your integrity, then, will determine whether the path is one of stress or one of joy.

Take a moment and look deep inside so that you can understand, as fully as possible, why you want to develop this part of your natural state of being. It is an important question to ask because from it other important value-based questions will arise.

Two Sacred Laws

In order for your intuitive awareness to strengthen and grow, it is imperative that you follow what I believe are two sacred laws of intuitive development. The first is *committing to your wisdom*, honoring and trusting your intuitive guidance whenever it comes to you and not dismissing it. In the process of learning to commit to your inner intuitive wisdom, you will occasionally not trust in yourself, as you probably already have from time to time. So now is the time to start. Take out your journal and write that you will follow this first sacred law: *You will commit to your intuitive wisdom, honoring and trusting whatever comes to you.*

The second sacred law is: *Live in the moment.* All you have is this moment, and then it is gone, only to be replaced by yet another. Live this moment as fully as you can. Do not place worry or burden within these precious moments; they are a distraction and they deplete your energy. There is a Buddhist insight that says, if you can't fix it, don't worry; if you can fix it, don't worry. This is wisdom worth following.

The magic of your intuition will seem to manifest and strengthen right before your eyes. It will change your life, especially if you apply these two sacred laws to your life and way of being. When you commit to your intuitive wisdom and make an effort to reside fully in the moment, you really can't make any mistakes. You are reaching deep inside yourself for your truth, and as a result your life will begin to unfold in a more sacred, intuitive, and satisfying manner. If you are not happy with the way your life is going, start trusting the deeper intuitive truth within you and you will effect the changes you desire. Commit to your wisdom instead of the thoughts or ideas that have been imposed on you by such external sources as your family or society.

Trusting your intuitive wisdom and being present in the moment will not, of course, mean life will be free of struggles and challenges, but it will mean you are living your truth as closely as you can. You will continue to learn, since that is the nature of your life as a human being—you are here to grow and evolve. However, the learning will be filled with more truth, wisdom, and joy. And life will become smoother—one of the truly pleasant aspects of developing yourself intuitively. Any challenges you encounter will seem to roll off your back. Your wisdom will direct your power. As a result, fear will diminish and at times disappear. As you learn to trust yourself, commit to your wisdom, and live in the moment, your intuitive abilities will continue to grow.

Developing your intuition connects you more intimately to all things. Intuition places you in the womb of co-creation with God, the planet, all living things, and the multitude of dimensions otherwise inaccessible to the five senses of your ordinary way of being. The power of your intuition will open you to the multidimensional universe. It takes you beyond what is probable in your life to what is possible. Then, as you practice and hone your abilities, you move beyond the world of possibilities and into the realm of potentiality.

There you will find the nonlocal mind and a fully expanded intuitive sense—a world in which there is no past, present, or future, since there is only one moment in time and space. This moment is a place where everything is knowable and tangible through your intuitive senses. It is a place where the life-force energy inside you is honored, where you are at peace knowing, in a deep bodily way, that you are one with the universe.

Varieties of Intuition

Some of the avenues through which universal information flows from the larger, primary source into your smaller, limited reality can shock or startle you, whereas others might be subtle and sublimely beautiful. But all are aspects of the same powerful conduit of intuition. The following stories illustrate some of the many different ways you might experience the power of intuition.

Often, intuition simply taps you on the shoulder and offers a helpful tip or warning. Jeanie came to see me in September one year. She was a healthcare professional with a highly developed intuition, but she was working too hard for others and ignoring her body's needs. I shared with her my concerns about her overloaded schedule and its effects on her immune system and body chemistry. My commentary was based on intuitive observations, the most prevalent being that energetic particles of cancer were beginning to develop in her electromagnetic field. They were forming around hip height, slightly left of center, and approximately four and a half feet away from her body.

I offered suggestions such as going to her conventional doctor, seeking out traditional Chinese medicine and homeopathy, and pursuing other avenues that could help relieve what was building in her field. Jeanie left the office and I did not hear from her until April of the following year. She shared with me that in January she seemed to get a cold from the inside out. I know that sounds strange, but I understood what she meant, and her energy indicated that the cancer was settling into her body.

One of the spiritual lessons for Jeanie was to pay attention to her own gift of intuition and listen to her body. I sensed the cancer's location and I knew it had just started to grow in her uterus. She needed to see her doctor. I shared this with her and told her to get in touch with what was going on inside her. She needed to do this in order to be her own advocate in what she was about to face.

I suggested that she ask her body and her spirit to show her a dream about what was happening in her body. That night she dreamed that cells were climbing up her body. She found herself on a dark battlefield in which soldiers from the same side were killing each other. The dream also revealed some energy of past abusive relationships. She awoke the next morning with a crystal-clear idea of what was happening in her body and called her doctor, who ran tests. Her intuitive diagnosis was confirmed.

She chose to jump on the treatment path of surgery, following her doctor's advice. She had a partial hysterectomy in which only the uterus was removed. She was cured. That was seven years ago. Jeanie is still a healthcare worker, and now she listens to her intuition with vigor, a balanced perspective, and gratitude.

As Jeanie's story shows, dreams are an important source of intuitive information. They often provide a clearer and more direct connection with your source of truth, especially since your active mind is resting and out of the way. Dreams may bring intuitive knowledge in the form of symbols or even whole scenarios concerning future events, loved ones, or aspects of your health and well-being.

My close friend Mary had a dream that again demonstrates the role of dreaming as a conduit of intuition. She dreamed that her daughter and son-in-law, who were living in South Africa, had died and a family debate ensued over where they would be buried. At three o'clock in the morning, she was awakened by the horror of this dream, hoping there was no connection between it and reality. Only three hours later, she received a phone call informing her that her daughter and son-in-law had been in a head-on auto accident, and her daughter had come so close to death that she had had an out-of-body experience. Mary's dream clearly demonstrated the existence of the transpersonal emotional fabric that interconnects us all and is accessible through intuition.

In a waking state, you might find that your intuition comes with a particular resonance in connection with specific events around you. Or an intuitive episode may be followed by a string of meaningful events. It may seem as if symbols, objects, and events are put in your path to guide you in a new direction or toward a new understanding. An underlying order starts to emerge that suggests an intelligence or power greater than your own that is actively helping you understand your role in the larger picture.

Susan, a student and client, shared a meaningful experience she had while participating in my Intuitive Therapeutics class. During the class, I guided students through an intuitively based auric field reading of one another. The task was simply to report to their partners the information they received as they intuitively scanned their classmates' energy. Scanning her partner's body, Susan saw bright red and yellow flashes of light in and around both of her partner's knees. In addition, she saw very dark blue energy embedded in her partner's shoulder that ran down her left arm. Her partner confirmed that she had chronic knee pain and that she had just contacted a chiropractor concerning shoulder and arm pain.

Confirmation of this variety happens every day for students and may even seem rather mundane. Such an affirmation, however, reveals the profound and beautiful truth of the intimate connection between the largest levels of the universe and the self. It is a marvelous fact of life that everyone can do this type of work to varying degrees, depending on intention and the desire to open and grow. Susan's child-like wonder at the implications of what she had just experienced amazed and thrilled her—she could intuitively see! To suddenly real-ize that intuition is deeply embedded in your being and that through it, you can be in touch with your source, is possibly one of the most satisfying results of exploring its power.

Becky had been a client for a few years and had been successful in honing her intuition with some of the exercises that are included in this book. She could sense when imbalances started to occur in her body. One day she called me because she had been feeling ill at ease and knew there was something going on in her body. She could intuitively feel it, but couldn't quite pin it down. I asked her if she had been experiencing a cold or cough. She confirmed that she had. I sensed virulent bacteria in the upper right lobe of her lung that I had not seen before, and sug-gested she see her doctor.

Becky does things quickly and at a top level. She immediately checked into the Mayo Clinic, where they indeed found unusual bacte-ria and prescribed antibiotics. Becky had been paying attention to her body's messages and stopped an illness before it got out of control.

Accessing Your Intuition

So many people tell me they would like to be able to see as I do. I usu-ally tell them that they, too, can access their intuitive information effectively once they find the way that comes to them most naturally and readily. Based on twenty years of experience teaching intuitive development, I have found that perhaps the most critical element is understanding how you naturally process information so that you can look in the right places for the doorway to your intuition. Without this element, many people find their intuitive growth stunted and their intuitive information distorted and weak.

Since all things in the universe are made of energy, the question is, "How do we sense this energy?" The first thing to realize is that there is a particular way in which you most easily access intuitive information. It is the way you most readily assimilate stimuli and articulate and act on them. Your intuitive means may be visual, auditory, empathic (also referred to as "kinesthetic"), or olfactory in nature. You might also access intuitive knowledge in what I call a perceptual way, by means of a sense of deep inner knowing. You may not see, hear, feel, or smell energy so much as know it when it comes to you.

Sheri, a student, once told me that the way she knows intuitive information is coming to her is that such thoughts seem to come into her awareness from the side of her body, whereas logical thoughts come to her straight on. As a result of understanding how intuitive insights come to her, Sheri was best able to pay attention to and access her intuition. This is but one example; we all have our own ways of receiving intuitive information. It may take some time and practice to discern the way in which you access yours, but your wellness and life's joy will reward your effort.

In order for you to gain an understanding of your preferred way of accessing your intuition, answer the following short questionnaire. Even if you already have a good idea of what your preference is—organizational, visual, auditory, empathic, olfactory, or perceptual—go through the questionnaire anyway; you will either be confirmed in your view or perhaps surprised to discover something new. In addition to the questionnaire, simply paying attention is an important way to discover your preferred intuitive channels. As you move through your daily life and experience more and more flashes of intuition, pay attention to the emotional, bodily, and mental sensations accompanying the intuitive information that is conveyed to you.

Intuitive Preference Questionnaire

Place a check mark beside any statement that fits you most of the time. Then enter the total number of checks at the end of each section and compare your totals with the key at the end of the questionnaire.

Organizational Style

____ I quickly and easily compute numbers in my head.

____ I enjoy figuring out abstract relationships between objects, people, and/or situations.

____ I love to follow and learn about the current trends in science.

____ I enjoy pondering "What if..." questions and often view the world from this perspective.

____ My mind searches for structures, patterns, sequences, or a logical and rational order to things and to life.

____ I enjoy reading about new technological discoveries and advances.

____ I think that a rational explanation exists for almost everything.

____ It is easy for me to think abstractly.

____ I can find flaws in others' reasoning and I enjoy engaging in debates.

____ I feel most comfortable when things are well organized.

____ **Total**

Visual Style

____ I have to see something in order to understand or remember it.

____ I am sensitive to colors and patterns.

____ I prefer to look at books and magazines with lots of illustrations.

____ I like to keep a visual record of my life; pictures of people, places, and events surround me and fill my home/office.

____ I can alter my inner visual perspective and see an object at both its microscopic and actual size.

____ My dreams tend to be vivid and in color.

____ I have a good sense of direction.

____ I use landmarks to orient myself.

____ I can easily see in my mind's eye people, places, or events whenever I hear a description or describe something to someone.

____ Sometimes I see flashes of color emanating from my hands, other people, or even plants and animals.

____ Total

Auditory Style

____ I often have a tune running through my head during the day.

____ I have a musical ear.

____ If I hear someone humming a tune, I pick it up easily.

____ I prefer listening to the radio or a CD to watching TV.

____ I have a good ear for accents and foreign languages.

____ I remember and understand things better if I hear them explained to me.

____ I often hear noises other people don't notice.

____ Sounds stimulate my thinking and imagination.

____ I receive information and guidance verbally in my mind.

____ Going beyond magical thinking, the songs that I hear in my head feel like guidance and messages that fit perfectly with my current situation.

____ Total

Empathic Style

____ I regularly participate in physical activities such as yoga, aerobics, dance, or sports.

____ I dislike sitting still for long periods of time.

____ I can feel the energy in a room as soon as I enter it.

____ My thinking and imagination are most stimulated when I am involved in a physical activity.

____ I both like to and need to spend a lot of time in nature.

____ I use a lot of gestures and other nonverbal cues when I talk.

____ I feel most connected to things when I can touch or feel them.

____ I can feel in my body the sensations that mirror what other people are feeling.

____ I have good physical coordination.

____ I learn most easily when I physically practice or act out something.

____ **Total**

Olfactory Style

____ I can smell sickness in people even before they show signs of an illness.

____ I like to sleep with the windows open.

____ I can smell things in my dreams.

____ I vividly remember the smells associated with events in my life.

____ I pick up smells other people don't notice.

____ When I get upset, I get sinus headaches or congestion.

____ Stuffy rooms make me nervous or uncomfortable.

____ I can identify even subtle spices in food using my sense of smell.

____ I am very sensitive to fragrances or strong scents.

____ **Total**

Perceptual Style

____ I get feelings of knowing that seem to arise from nowhere—and end up being true.

____ I can sense when something is not right.

____ I can meet someone and instantly know things about them.

____ I know what kind of mood my children, spouse, or work peers are in before I see them.

____ A person will come to my mind and a day or two later I will be surprised to see or speak with them.

____ I know if something good is going to happen.

____ I have an uncanny sense of direction.

____ People I know and even strangers open up to me and tell me their problems.

____ **Total** (Four or more checks in this category means you have an intuitive perceptual preference.)

Now compare your total number of checks for each style. Your preferred intuitive style is the style that has the most checks. If you ended up with a tie between styles, it simply means that you have more than one way to access intuition.

This questionnaire should give you a clearer picture of your own preference for responding to energetic stimuli and accessing intuitive information. Knowing your preference lets you begin to understand where your intuitive strengths are and how you can best tap into them.

A word about the empathic intuitive style: Empathic-oriented people access intuitive information through their bodies. As a result, they sometimes find it difficult to be in crowded, noisy places where they are affected by a lot of energy. Moreover, empathic people who are continually in stressful situations usually either have weight fluctuations or hold onto weight. They automatically layer on fat to protect themselves emotionally and protect certain vital organs. If, for example, you are empathic and have been overworking or are stressed, you might notice you have added a little extra padding to the back of your waist; this is the result of an attempt to protect your adrenal glands, which are affected by stress you hold in your body.

Note also that the questions concerning the organizational style are intended to help you identify how much time you spend in your logical, or rational, mind. There is nothing wrong with using your rational mind, but in connection with intuitive development, it is better to shelve this part of yourself until you have honed your intuitive skills enough so that you can incorporate the use of the logical mind at the appropriate time. Intuition and intellect can work side by side. First, however, the intuitive pathway needs to be cleared and accessible in order for that information to come forward. Then the intellect can put the intuitive pieces of the puzzle together if need be.

You might have realized that, like many of us, you have more than one effective pathway to your intuition. In my case, for example, I use my seeing, feeling, hearing, and knowing pathways to do my work. Sometimes the pathway I use depends on the person I am reading, or my environment. Don't get hung up on using one style or another; just ride along with where you are now and know that you will probably add more pathways as you practice and develop your intuition.

Intuitive preferences may last for a certain duration and then change as your life progresses. For example, currently you may be visually oriented; six months from now, however, you may experience a shift and become more empathic. This change usually results from the development of your intuitive ability, although personality maturation can also contribute to the change. Use the questionnaire as a launching pad, a guide to some of your preferred routes to accessing your intuition, but bear in mind that your tendencies will likely evolve as you change and grow.

Honor Your Individual Preferences

Many students find the questionnaire and the discovery of the variety of possible preferences helpful, as it gives them permission to be who they are and lets them know that they don't have to be visual in order to work intuitively.

When I was lecturing at a convention in Tucson, Arizona, a situation arose that illustrates that each of us accesses intuition differently and that we often feel insecure about speaking our intuitive truth. After my lecture, the usual group of warm-hearted souls was waiting for some personal time with me. I noticed one woman hanging back, and she was the last person with whom I spoke. Mary was a nurse in an intensive care unit at a local hospital. She related to me that she smelled the fragrance of flowers around certain patients when they were about to cross over from this life into the next. She also noticed foul odors around some patients just prior to their taking a sudden turn for the worse. Mary touchingly shared how she could sense all of these things and could therefore act more appropriately toward her patients, taking care of them with greater understanding based on her olfactory intuition. I thought that all the patients who were touched by this woman had been truly graced and blessed. A nurse as sensitive to her patients' needs and situations as Mary is clearly the type of nurse I would want attending me.

This illustrates that you don't have to be visually oriented to access your intuitive information. Mary was certainly tuned in the way that was most natural for her. It is important to realize that society has set forth the myth, "I'll believe it when I see it." As an intuitive individual you don't have to accept that myth any longer. Following cosmic law, the myth might more accurately be stated the other way around: Believe it and then you'll see it.

Another example of intuitive preference comes from a charming and warm student of mine named Sasha. She had worked as a computer analyst, but after completing the first-level training program of Intuitive Therapeutics, she timidly hung out her healer's shingle. She is continuing her intuitive training in order to be the best she can be in her new career.

Sasha hears the various tones at which the chakras resonate. Receiving her intuitive information in the most natural way for her, she can detect imbalances in a person's system by hearing his body's sour tones, and in that way she knows where to adjust his energy. As with Sasha and other intuitives, committing to your intuitive wisdom, no matter what your way of accessing it might be, allows you to make accurate assessments and facilitate your own or a client's healing and awareness.

Through my travels, by exchanging stories I have found that many people have had the same experiences I have had. We have all been receiving intuitive information our entire lives. The unfortunate thing is that most of us have been afraid to share it. You don't have to be afraid anymore! Be discerning, certainly, but trust and honor your intuitive wisdom. If you don't own this wondrous component, your energetic system will clog, which can cause dissonance, misalignment, and possibly even disease. Listening to and acting on your intuition honors a wonderful, innate part of who you are.

I'll never forget the look on one woman's face in class when she finally understood that it was okay for her to receive her intuitive guidance in the form of just knowing a condition or situation. For years Karen thought that because she didn't see images or hear intuitive information—she simply knew—she was wrong. Karen is a perceiver, yet for all those years she didn't trust herself or commit to her wisdom. She was relieved and grateful to gain a new understanding of the ability she knew she had but had never given herself permission to use. After this realization, her intuitive development was swift.

These few simple stories illustrate that we all have different pathways through which we harvest the vast amount of divine intuitive information that is available to us. Trust the way in which your intuitive wisdom comes to you. You simply need to find your source and the conduit through which it passes. Keeping in mind that your pathway might be different from everyone else's, permit yourself to grow naturally toward your development. We are all different and move at our own pace. By honoring the way in which intuitive wisdom can most easily be gathered and acted upon, we create a better quality of life and wellness for ourselves and everyone around us.

Developing Your Intuitive Awareness Mindfully

Now that you recognize that you are intuitive and have discovered your intuitive style preference, it is time to understand what may transpire as you develop your intuition and access your health wisdom. Remember that life is a process, not an event. The same applies to intuitive development. As you progress, there will definitely be milestones; nonetheless, for the most part your intuitive development will unfold more or less continually. Synchronicities, flashes of illumination, moments of doubt, and wondrous as well as subtle experiences all interrelate in a complex system of learning and growth that constitutes an important component of your daily practice.

Intuitive development is closely tied to mindfulness. Being mindful is awakening without attachment to the myriad stimuli that surround all things. The concept of mindfulness comes from deep in the belly of Buddhism. Behaving mindfully is being awake to and aware of the subtleties around oneself, and therefore having the ability to respond rather than react to them.

We humans use only a small percentage of our brains' capacity. Consequently, it could be assumed that we are moving through our lives aware of only a small portion of what is truly happening around us. By parting the curtains of the window to our world just a fraction, we allow only a tiny ray of illumination into our minds.

Mindfulness will open the doors to your soul and mind through which intuition can walk. It has been my experience that the cultivation of intuition and mindfulness go hand in hand—they are opposite sides of the same coin. It is thus vital that you practice mindfulness to develop your intuitive capacity. Pay attention. Be awake. As you cultivate mindfulness, your intuition will necessarily grow, and at the same time, as your intuition develops and builds, you will become more mindful of your environment. As you develop your intuitive abilities, you will gain a greater understanding of the interconnectedness of all things and their systems of cycles. You will shed the limited perspective of consciousness that perceives duality and a three-dimensional perspective as the only true, hard reality. Instead, your journey in the development of intuition will guide you to the absolute and ultimate way of being.

How Much You Practice Determines Your Progress

Intuitive development can be understood to rest on what I have developed as the fourfold Intuitive Healing model: 1) practice meditation and stillness; 2) learn to consciously move energy through your body with energy medicine techniques and practices such as qigong, tai chi, and yoga; 3) apply the skills you learn in these first two levels in everyday life; 4) experience the effortlessness that will become part of your life. As a model it is represented like this:

Practice meditation and stillness
Consciously move energy
Apply skills every day
Experience effortlessness

Natural protocols that lead to understanding and inner wisdom are a major aspect of your intuitive development. These protocols, which you will call upon every day both formally and informally, are a spiritual means of taking care of yourself. This spiritual means may consist of, but is not limited to, such activities as prayer, meditation, physical exercise, visualization exercises, good nutrition, and proper speech toward yourself and others. The exercises in this book will assist you in developing this aspect of your daily practice. It is up to you to decide which protocols you will follow and exactly what you want to include in your spiritual tool kit.

Of course, your daily practice depends on the development of discipline. Discipline will assist you in creating the space in your life for your practice. The discipline you cultivate expresses honor and loyalty to yourself and your chosen path. It also relates to your devotion—devotion to your spirit, body, mind, and your spiritual source.

Your progress will be equal to the quality of your spiritual practice. There is simply no substitute for a well thought out, motivated practice for developing intuition.

My students and clients over the years have found success through applicable techniques, not just theory. You have to put a practice or technique into your body to really know what you are doing, and that experience builds trust, faith, and the ability to own your power. As you develop yourself intuitively and spiritually, it is important that you apply what you are practicing to your daily life, especially to the seemingly mundane tasks.

There is a story of a young monk who was a newcomer to a particular monastery. Every morning the monks would gather at the central well to bathe. On this young monk's first morning at the well, he asked an older monk if the water was cold. Without saying a word, the older monk picked up a bucket of the well water and dumped it over the young monk's body. The wise old monk knew that firsthand experience would give the young monk a greater understanding than simply being told the answer. The important point is this: If you know but you do not do, you don't really know.

Your single most powerful tool is your innate wisdom, your intuition. The only way to strengthen it is by practicing it.

Recommended Exercises

Intuitive Shopping
The Power of Movement

3
Mastering Your Mind

The ceaseless chatter of the mind is an experience we can all relate to. The challenge is to master the chatter, which seems to spin out of control at times, and master the mind—literally and energetically dissolve the chattering mind into a state of emptiness. I experienced this emptiness when I was in the throes of my near-death experience. I entered into a state of emptiness described in the Heart Sutra, a prayer from Buddhism that describes a mind free from attachments. I had "no eyes, no ears, no tongue, no body, no mind." I had "no life, no death, and also no extinction of them." I also experienced a consciousness rising and falling within—what I can only describe as a dark, velvety soup of universal consciousness. There was no fear, no attachment to the life I had left, nor any attachment to what lay in front of me. I was simply empty.

It has been both my experience and observation that obtaining that state of emptiness while holding the form of a physical body and remaining immersed in your life takes practice and is indeed an art. Developing the practice and the art of easing your mind's grip over your life is a valuable aim, especially when it comes to reading your energy to bring about healing. As you begin to use your intuition for self-healing, your mind needs some direction and support to become still so you can receive intuitive information. When I do healing facilitation with others I know that it is not helpful to let my mind run amok while working with another's energy. Remember, energy is a by-product of consciousness, and when I speak of working with energy, I am referring to working with other people's consciousness and the thought forms that weave themselves in and out of their present state.

It is not a good idea, therefore, for me to have focused thoughts about myriad other things while I am energetically working in someone's liver that may or may not be filled with disease. It is absolutely critical for anyone doing healing facilitation to stay present, for the client's sake as well as the facilitator's. Learning mindfulness-based meditation provides skillful means by which you can hold your intuitive focus on the task at hand and not be carried away by your mind's chatter. Generally, a state of centeredness and calm, even in the midst of chaos, is the desired place to be.

Understanding Thought Forms

In the process of becoming enlightened, you will come to understand the source and activity of your mind, particularly its thought forms. Thought forms create your reality. Like prayers or mantras, they are charged with energetic levels of consciousness and certain emotional essences. These emotional charges are catalysts for manifestation.

When I scan someone's body, I am looking for disorder, imbalance, and disease. But I'm also focusing on the thought forms inside the cellular structure of the body, as well as those held within the energetic field surrounding it. The location, directional movement, and emotional charge of the thought forms indicate the extent of the imbalance, disorder, or disease. These thought forms are the chatter that subconsciously directs emotions, behavior, biochemistry, and a host of other aspects of human existence.

You can learn to perceive thought forms no matter how you access your intuitive wisdom. A characteristic of my way of accessing intuitive information is that my seeing can be molecularly oriented. This orientation allows me to intuitively track the directional movement of a disease, such as cancer, and perceive thought forms either in the body or in the surrounding energy field. To track something of this nature I tune in to the intelligence that resides within both healthy cells and diseased ones. Within that intelligence I will intuitively see and hear the "intention" of what the cell's intelligence holds. Whether it is a cell or the energetic particles in the field, there is a sense of which way is it headed, whether it is growing or receding.

When I look through my mind's eye at someone's energy field, I see a kind of aqueousness of consciousness surrounding the person. All your thought forms creating your current reality and bringing together new constructs float in and around this field that mantles your physical body.

I can discern where someone is on a consciousness level by looking at the rate of vibration of a person's thought forms within both the aqueous or energy field and the cellular structure of the body. Inconsistencies appear as light and energy fluctuations in the various layers of the body, with shuttering and spiking motions. These reactions demonstrate in the electromagnetic field, in the body, in areas that are hiding falsehoods, as well as in the light energy around the cells. People may say certain things about where they are and what they want in their lives, yet their lives don't seem to match their words. Why is this? It is because the thought forms residing in their energy fields do not match what they are saying. It is not that they do not desire certain things (to lose weight, make more money, or be kinder or more mindful); it is that an inconsistency exists between the present thought forms and those that would create the desired reality. This inconsistency often creates inconsistent behaviors as well.

Limiting thought forms can result from enculturation, imprinting, or the influence of what other people say to you or tell you to do. That is why it is important to understand how your energy, your consciousness, runs through your body. There are numerous exercises in the back of this book that will help you better understand how energy moves through you. Do you think it is valuable to understand how your partner's energy affects you? Or how the energy at your office runs through your energy centers? Such awareness will allow you to discern what is yours and what isn't, and if it isn't, whether you want to hang onto it. Do the thoughts that run through your mind serve you? That is an important question to ask yourself from time to time, but especially when you catch a thought that makes you feel out of balance or unwell.

The work you do as you move toward enlightenment will allow you to identify more clearly the thought forms that create your reality. Formulating what you desire to be more abundant in your life and holding that thought form above all others will create that which you seek.

Since I have been able to practice and hone my intuitive skills in this manner, I know you can also develop your ability to perceive phenomena at this level. The aim for all of us, healing facilitators and those with whom we work, is ultimately to move beyond the level of phenomena, beyond limiting thought forms that restrict us to a particular reality, toward an unattached, unlimited consciousness, which will bring us closer to inner peace.

Mastering your mind to bring about wellness takes time, discipline, self-awareness, persistence, kindness to yourself and others, and a deep awareness of the universal love always belonging to you. You can be free of your mind's limiting beliefs and your body's disorders, diseases, and misalignments if you commit to your wisdom and allow it to propel you forward, however gradually. Simply hold the awareness of unlimited consciousness that is naturally within you. Remember that you are an illuminating ray that shines from and is connected to the macrocosm, the body of God, and the one pure universal mind.

You're Not Crazy, You're Becoming Enlightened!

As you make progress mastering your mind, guided by the wisdom of whatever spiritually based path you have chosen, you will at times face abrupt changes. These sudden shifts in consciousness can sometimes throw you that all-powerful cosmic curveball, making you question what you are doing and just where you are going with all of this.

We've all experienced it. There you are, walking along on your personally fashioned yellow brick road to enlightenment, when suddenly chaos strikes. Old, crazy thoughts swirl in and out of your consciousness like tornadoes. What makes it worse is that these are the very thoughts that have beaten you down, shamed you, cursed you, and thrown you into a repressed or depressed state in the past. They are the thoughts that you have been so dedicated to eradicating from your life. You know them—the ones that say:

- I'm never going to get out of this situation.
- I'm fat.
- I'm ugly.
- I can't possibly take care of myself.
- I'm not allowed to be proud of myself.
- I'll never make enough money to keep my head above water.

- I'll never be able to quit my job and do work that honors my spirit.

- I'm not really a healer.

- I should just stay in this unhappy marriage.

- I'll never be able to make the changes I want in my life.

- I'm not smart enough and there isn't enough time or money to go after what I want.

- I have to take care of others before I think about myself.

- I will never escape my suffering.

On and on they go, rattling around in your consciousness, loud, ugly, and relentless.

But the good news is that when these thoughts arise, it means that they're lifting away from your body's cellular memory, as well as from the old constructs of your mind that created the reality. The work you have been doing to master your mind is getting results! You are succeeding at releasing those thoughts and constructs, and you are in the process of changing the binding reality that has kept you shackled; you are fully engaged in creating your new reality.

It's not always easy to see this when cascades of thought forms are pounding you once again, but know that they are coming squarely at you to challenge you and make sure that you are really ready to let go of them. They are there to say good-bye to you. It is important to recognize this period as a natural phase in the consciousness-raising process. Engage your mindfulness skills and watch the thoughts rise and descend within your mind. They are just thoughts. For instance, if you think of an abusive partner, your thought is not that person; it is merely a thought. Let the thoughts go, with love and blessings for the lessons they have bestowed upon you.

Many events from my own life and from my clients' and students' lives have shown me that when old thought forms emerge this is usually what is happening. Once I had a young woman named Vivian in my office describing her struggles. She had just taken a job in another city and was at home with her husband only on weekends. For the past several months, she had been positioning herself to leave her husband and her marriage. She had, seemingly out of thin air, created a new job for herself. She had also secured a place to live with some friends in her new city.

During the few weeks prior to these changes, her experiences with her husband began to shift. Normally violent at times, her husband was suddenly being nicer to her, which led her to doubt her decision to leave him. "If he's being so nice," she reasoned to herself, "and we're getting along now, why not stay?" Other, similar thoughts began to arise in her. She also knew, however, that her husband's temper was being chemically sedated. Still, the thoughts of staying kept surfacing, strongly and steadily, whirling around in her mind and causing her to feel confused. After all, she had been holding her intention and attention on leaving and creating a new life for herself—a life of peace, spirituality, and freedom. Her current experience with her new job and a safe haven to live in was demonstrating to her the ease with which her new life was being created. I could see Vivian's confusion, not only in her speech but also in her auric field while we talked.

Exasperated, she explained that although she had been doing her spiritual work—meditations, prayers, affirmations—in the past few weeks the thoughts that she had been attempting to transform had suddenly begun hounding her even more relentlessly than before. She said that since she was having these thoughts of "giving in and staying" so forcefully and so often, maybe she should; maybe they were some divine guidance to stay. But her gut, her body, was still screaming, "Go!"

I assured her that neither her divine guidance nor anyone else's would ever suggest or demand through thought forms that a person stay in an abusive or oppressive situation or relationship. Such suggestions are not divinity at work; they arise from the ego at a stage of karma-releasing growth. Moreover, the tangible, rapid creation of new circumstances—her new job and place to stay—demonstrated support for the new reality she was creating. All of this illustrated that a path was indeed opening, allowing her to step into a new realm of freedom. Those thoughts of "giving up and staying" were the very ones that had kept her in her marriage for so long. These thought forms were mechanisms her mind used to keep her from moving forward with her life, implanted in her by the karmic relationship between herself and her husband. The re-emerging thoughts were displacing the personal perspective of her self-esteem, which the relationship's abusive nature had whittled away. Her task for growth was to release them and see herself in a new way.

I began to smile as Vivian bemoaned the fact that she just couldn't understand how she could be doing all this work and still experience these thoughts so incessantly. She stopped mid-sentence and asked what I was smiling about. I assured her that all her spiritual practice was working. The tenacity of old thought forms also demonstrated that they were on their way out and would very soon be gone: It was their last farewell. Their suddenness and strength showed that she had been doing all the right things. She had created a new set of thought forms, reframing and transforming the old ones.

You are the architect of your reality, building your life through a variety of thought forms. Understanding the architectural components, along with the methods you use to dismantle and reconstruct your reality, is also important. Realize that when you want to remodel and rebuild, you have to create new space within your body and both your subconscious and conscious minds.

In Vivian's case, she had been dismantling her thought forms and her life was being remodeled. The old thought forms were on their way out—out of her mind, out of her body—and their exit, the way they could express to her that they were leaving, was to storm out of her body and her body's energy through her mind. Her task was to recognize that since she was so dedicated to her path of self-transformation, these old, negative thoughts were coming up to say good-bye to her. Her other task was to let them go as graciously as possible. Indeed, these two tasks belong to all of us.

As you step toward your own enlightenment, other things can occur that drive you crazy. Things get misplaced or lost—including you! Once I was traveling to the post office, a trip I take at least five times a week. At this particular time in my life, however, I was in the middle of a nine-week meditation practice of periodic silence. I say periodic because I was still seeing clients and teaching, but the rest of the time I kept silent and alone, working on specific meditations and visualizations to lift my own consciousness. As I drove along my usual route, suddenly everything that I knew as familiar no longer was; I had absolutely no recognition of where I was.

I knew that I was on my way to the post office. I knew that I had just turned onto the street I usually take. Nonetheless, all the things along this segment of the trip were strange and oddly unfamiliar. Now, this happens to some extent to all of us occasionally. But the time I remained in this state of unrest was rather long by my usual standards, five minutes or so. I watched as an aspect of my mind began to grow more and more uncomfortable. Then I remembered the intention behind my current practice: to raise my consciousness. I realized that this momentary loss of reality, although lasting only five minutes, was an indication that my work was effective. I settled into the fact that although I had no cognitive clue as to where I was, on some level I understood where I was going simply out of habit, and that I only needed to accept what was happening. Laughing, I realized that for a few moments I had been able to let go of the hard boundaries of my old reality, even its physical form and manifestation.

You might find, too, that you lose the tools that assist you in moving your physical body through your world: your keys, driver's license, day planner, and things of that nature. They will suddenly disappear for a time and then reappear, seemingly by magic. When I went through my divorce, I kept losing my driver's license. I could only laugh about it, because I knew it meant that I was changing the way I moved through the world. My name and direction were changing, so the temporary loss of my driver's license was not a surprise; in fact, I saw it as a positive sign.

Incidents such as these may or may not happen to you, or they may have already occurred and you just assumed you were losing your mind! But if you are in the midst of a practice, most likely you are shifting consciousness and not experiencing problems related to neurological or cognitive functionality. (Please note that I am not making light of neurological or cognitive disorders that can cause biochemical shifts in the body and alterations in the mind. Should they occur, seek appropriate medical assistance.) As you break through portions of your seemingly hard reality, remember that all the things around you are just molecules that agree, for whatever reason or mode of attraction, to hang out and coagulate as certain forms and structures.

Years ago, I was doing some hands-on healing work with a woman in my office. During the session, I was moving my hand about four inches or so above her left calf and was deeply involved in the process of shifting the molecular structure of her leg's energy when something rather odd occurred. To my shock, a portion of her calf physically shifted right before my eyes. As I looked at her left leg, I could plainly see her foot, ankle, and knee; but the midsection of her calf had turned into what I can only describe as a patch of energy consisting of grayish-white light particles, floating and moving very rapidly in current-like patterns. The sudden transformation of her calf into what I believe we are all actually made of surprised me so much that I jumped back. The whole experience lasted for maybe no more than ten seconds. Nonetheless, I shifted my thinking that day regarding what was real and what wasn't. Because of that experience, I dedicated myself even more diligently to my work with molecular structure and its nature in connection with healing, energy medicine, and the creation of reality.

Other things can occur because of the success of your spiritual practice as your reality changes. Relationships change, and by this I mean your relationships with everything and everyone. Relationships naturally change along with your inner relationship with yourself and your God source, whatever form that takes for you. Your relationships with your home, family, and friends will inevitably change. Even your relationship with such things as your clothes will change. It will move beyond the "I can't find anything to wear" statement arising primarily from an ego state to the "I can't find anything to wear" that expresses the fact that it all looks foreign and no longer seems to fit your body. For when you are involved in your spiritual practice, even if you are sitting still in thought, prayer, affirmation, and meditation, your body's structure will change. A deep practice brings about changes that reflect its depth. The clothes in your closet will simply not fit for awhile. You might find, too, that the colors, styles, and coordinates you were attracted to no longer seem to complement you and your new state of energetic being. This development will not necessarily mean that you have to go out and buy new things; just be prepared for the altered perspective so you won't be shocked by changes in your relationship to your living environment and your belongings.

All the objects and people in your life have resonated with your energetic state and consciousness level. Your intention, attention, and newly created thought forms will change the vibration of your molecular structure. It is therefore natural that some of the relationships that you have resonated with in the past will not feel the same or even good anymore.

Other events that indicate that you are shifting might make you think you're losing your connectedness; and, in a way, you are, but only for a time. I know a gifted young woman, for example, who asked for my assistance in discovering the ways in which she communicated with others via her intuition. Lauren was very gifted in seeing, hearing, and knowing; yet, at the time, she was unsure of how to articulate her information. She had called to make an appointment and talk about what she had been going through, and in her message, because her regular phone line was not working at the time, she gave me several different phone numbers by which to reach her. I tried several times to reach her using the numbers she had given me, but to no avail. I saw her mother a few weeks later and asked her to relay that I had tried unsuccessfully to call Lauren. I mentioned that I thought it was funny that her daughter was having trouble with her telephones—her mode of communication—just as she was also struggling with communicating with her inner guidance and with others.

When things like this happen to you, lighten up; don't take it all so seriously. Life can be tough, but your attitude—your thought forms—will either congest or clear your path. It's up to you. Oh, and Lauren? Currently both her intuitive gifts and phones are working just fine.

Don't be surprised or afraid when your outer reality demonstrates the changes occurring in your innermost self. That is the nature of nature. I often ask students how their meditation is going. I get all kinds of responses: confused, scattered, highly structured and ritualized, nonexistent, etc. I then ask them to think about how their lives are going. They are amazed to discover that their current life's structure mirrors their meditation—or is it the other way around? A still mind is a still life; a chattering, chaotic mind is a—well, you get the picture.

As you move forward on your journey, you will come to a time in your life when you will not have to dial up another psychic hotline or anyplace else to discover what your future and health will be. Simply look into your mind and your energetic field. There you will discover where your thoughts are, where they are going, and at what speed they are traveling. All will indicate your future. If you don't like what you see, feel, hear, or know, change your thought forms.

Developing Self-Discipline and Patience

The art of developing self-discipline and patience is like many other pursuits: Your progress will be equal to your practice. And as a component of personal spiritual development, it is an art you alone must take responsibility for as you move toward enlightenment and liberation. Being committed to your path and your intuitive wisdom will create the space in which discipline can occur. It is an obvious result. When you see the subtle benefits of this making a difference in your life, you will become more disciplined in setting aside some time for your spiritual practice.

You might find that laziness sometimes gets in the way of your desire to be disciplined and achieve your goals. When you are lazy, you are in effect not committed to yourself and you doubt your ability to do whatever task you would like to accomplish. Laziness can also lead to complaining, speaking ill of others, or putting blame where it does not belong. Complaining and blaming others actually displaces doubts about your abilities and a lack of commitment to yourself onto an external source. Pull those thought forms back inside and be accountable to yourself.

Laziness is also caused by allowing yourself to be distracted, usually by negative thoughts or actions. Understanding and seeing the good in yourself and in the world around you, realizing that there is a source greater than yourself, will help with this kind of laziness.

It is easier to develop good characteristics such as discipline and patience when you think about their benefits and positive aspects. For example, when you realize that discipline can relieve the suffering in your life, you are more inclined to practice it, and you will find new thoughts beginning to shift the old thought forms out of existence. It is important to have the awareness to catch the wave of an impulse as it arises within you; that impulse will lead to action and then generate motivation. People often say that they are not motivated to do something when they are actually missing or ignoring the impulse that comes from the intuitive cue to exercise, meditate, eat healthfully, etc. Catch the impulse. Act on it. Motivation will generate while you are doing the task and success will certainly follow. This series of events supports and solidifies discipline.

Loving yourself "right where you are" and holding this positive and helpful thought toward others is uplifting and generates patience and loving kindness. Set your mind's course on feeling and knowing these ideals deeply, then demonstrate them in kind and beneficial ways toward others. Regularly holding such thoughts will give you a happy life; you will find your pathway to liberation and peace. Manifest these thoughts through the personal talents, gifts, and resources that Spirit has given you, holding enlightenment for others and yourself as a goal. A clear path will open before you.

Realizing that we are all one will help you find patience and take you to a more peaceful place where it will not be so difficult to be disciplined about your life. Knowing that patience is the antidote to anger and underlying sadness allows you to simply respond to, rather than react to, aggression or negativity from others; it can also help you bring patience into your life. Understanding and gratitude also foster patience.

I have a friend named Bob with whom, at one time in my life, I spent a lot of time. He had a kind heart but, because of his life experiences, it was shadowed with anger and distrust. We were on an adventure in the desert one day when we came upon a beautiful and sacred bird—a Red-tailed Hawk—that had been killed in the road.

We stopped and took the bird into the desert and gave it a burial according to sacred traditions I had learned along my path. A day or two later while we were driving in the city, Bob told me that the experience of honoring the bird in that sacred way was the first time he had ever felt gratitude.

I was taken aback. His comment provoked more curiosity on my part than judgment toward him. It was hard for me to grasp that he honestly believed he had never experienced gratitude before. We talked further, and through our conversation it became clear to me that having gratitude in your life, which expresses an affirmation and acceptance of life as it is, allows you to let go of what you think life is supposed to be like. It allows you to be free and let others be free as well. Gratitude dissolves anger, sadness, distrust, and jealousy because it opens your heart to the expansiveness of experience. In this way, it fosters patience for yourself and others.

Make Time for Meditation and Prayer

Meditation and prayer are two of the most important ways to calm the mind and adhere to a spiritual practice. But many people complain that meditation is difficult or simply impossible for them. They think that since they cannot immediately still their minds, they are not meditating correctly. Just calming the body is difficult enough for many. Our culture has programmed us with an express lane mentality: Not only do people feel that they need to do it right, but they also put added pressure on themselves to do it quickly.

The truth is that in the beginning, meditation is simply letting the mind do what it will. Your task is to just be the observer and pay attention to how your mind processes and operates. One of the subtle pearls of a meditation practice is that you will understand the tendencies of your mind as you sit in your practice and observe. It may not be reasonable to expect to achieve a state of calm if you do not understand the state of your mind as it is now. Every thought you have rises in the mind and sinks back into it, only to be replaced in your consciousness by yet another thought.

Similarly, making time to connect and ask for help on your spiritual path is vital for creating balance in your being. It is a wise person who takes time out to pray, to ask God, Brahma, Great Spirit, Buddha, his soul, or the universal life energy, "What's up?" You know that when you are upset, chemicals flood your body. Likewise, when you are calm, peaceful, and relaxed, chemicals flood your body as well. Thus, your body is constantly being affected by different physiological (and energetic) responses, depending on which way your emotional pendulum is swinging at the time. When stress-activated chemicals pour into your bloodstream, muscles, and organ tissues, it is a good time to reverse those negative effects on your body by easing your mind. And one way of doing this is through prayer. It is not my place to tell you how to pray or what to pray for; those are deeply personal matters. But I do urge you to use this tool to get closer to the power that already resides within you.

Once I was giving a lecture and sharing the stage with a dear friend and a brilliant woman, Kathy Hanoseck, who has assisted many people in her successful fundraising efforts for nonprofits. Kathy took the stage first and was talking about her life's journey and gave an example of one of her favorite prayers. When things get tough in her life, her prayer is, "Aw, come on, God!!" The audience roared. What a great prayer!

Many years ago, when I was dealing with learning how to manage all the colors and energy I was seeing around people, I stood on a hilltop in southeastern Ohio, tears streaming from my eyes, yelling at God, "I want to know who I am and how to offer that in my service to others!" I got a little indignant with God in those days. I guess I figured that since I had gone from life to death to life again, what the heck could I lose by demanding what I wanted? And you know what? I have found that when I mix emotions with my prayers, the manifestation process happens really fast.

We have all experienced the power of prayer, whether we recognize it or not. Just do it. Pray. Stay humble. Question, yell, cry, and smile at the Gods above and ask for what you need, want, and desire. You just have to let those in the ether know what you want, pack a bit of emotion behind it, and move your thoughts and thought forms into alignment with your desires. Then stand back, watch, and be grateful!

People often ask me what I think their calling is. I cannot tell you what your calling is, but I can offer this suggestion: Your calling generates feelings in your heart, not in your gut. If the body sensations that your passion, your inner calling, generate in your heart, you are on target. You can wrestle with it in your gut, but its source is in the heart. If your heart yearns, but the sensations are stronger in your gut, you are off target.

Finding Support

Along your spiritual path you may encounter dark nights of the soul when you feel lost, powerless, and alone in the world. If you experience any of these feelings, take a piece of paper and write the following three words in this order:

- Trust
- Faith
- Power

Put this piece of paper where you can see it all the time—on your refrigerator, your computer monitor, the bathroom mirror, or anyplace in your house that calls to you (remember to use your intuition, even in such seemingly simple situations). Look at the words for a moment. If you feel power—not power over someone or something but empowered—you will own and feel secure in your concept of self. If you feel power in this way, you will automatically have faith—faith in yourself, faith in God, faith in what you are doing. Further, if you have power and faith, you will have trust—trust that the outcome of all things will be for your highest good. You will also trust in the universal support system that weaves its way throughout nature and life itself.

Conversely, if you don't trust in God, in yourself, in the oneness of all, you won't have faith that all will be well. And a lack of faith will most likely cause you to also feel powerless. So the next time you feel powerless or lack faith or trust, look at those three words in order, then do your spiritual practice, whatever it may be. Go to the woods, the ocean, or someplace else in nature and observe the universal oneness that connects us all. Draw power from watching a river or feeling the wind, snow, rain, or sunshine on your face. Lie belly-down on the land and absorb the power of Mother Earth as she too breathes in and out in her own way. Draw strength from your spiritual source, your family, or your friends.

If there is no external source from which you can draw, draw from the most fundamental source there is: the power that sleeps inside you. Close your eyes and focus your attention on your heart space. Feel the power inside shifting and churning. Through the experience of feeling something greater than yourself moving within your own physical body, a belief will form. It will form because you cannot deny what you have experienced inside yourself. You have felt the movement of life-force energy greater than yourself. Connect that life force inside you with your environment, and so understand the experience of oneness. As you do this, faith and trust will once more grace your life and you will feel empowered.

We've all experienced feeling quite alone—even in a crowd, a marriage, or a family. It is a feeling that seems to have nothing to do with where we are. Despite this universal experience, the fact is, we truly are not alone. There is a universal support system always holding us in some manner, whether we are aware of it or not.

Once I was sitting at the edge of a pool noticing the undulations of the water and the light and shadows as they danced across the bottom of the pool. The water and the moving light and shadows supported each other's existence. I found the image mesmerizing and I was lost in the moment.

Suddenly someone dove into the pool, shattering the gentle orchestration of water, light, and shadow. Chaos took over, but I sat there observing how, even though the water and its counterparts were disrupted, there was still a strong sense of unity, of support within the chaos. Slowly, without forgetfulness of their place in the order of life, the water, light, and shadow all came back to their calmer, undulating rhythm.

This experience demonstrated to me what I had observed in my own life's struggles. No matter what chaotic scene may be playing out, there is always a support system that balances and maintains the ordered cycles of life. When I demonstrate patience, faith, and trust in that system of support, I connect with the process of how all things maintain an innate sense of balance no matter what is transpiring. My job and yours is to gather grace during our chaotic times, always remembering the universal support system that underlies any confusion or disruption.

Recommended Exercises

Releasing Mind Chatter
Calming the Mind Through Breath

4

Getting to Know Your Energy Blueprint

In this chapter and throughout the book I often use the word "energy." When I speak of energy, I refer to two distinct qualities. First, energy is a by-product of consciousness; it is the demonstration of consciousness in a denser but still subtle form. Second, energy is more palpable than consciousness. For instance, when someone says something to you and you suddenly feel goose bumps or sourness in your stomach, you are feeling her consciousness physically as energetic sensations in your body. I call these "energetic impacts." Energetic impacts stimulate both your neurological and biochemical systems, consequently affecting the grosser levels of matter in your body—muscles, organ tissues, and bone structure. The exercises contained in this book will help you feel energy; but for now, I simply want you to be aware that what you are feeling are levels of consciousness—thought forms—that reside in and around your physical body.

In your body, you have an interconnected system of subtle lines and vortices of energy that both emanate from and support the denser molecular matter of your physical body. These lines or channels of energy are called *nadis* (NA-deez) in the Ayurvedic system of medicine of India. The vortices where the energetic channels converge to support the internal and external structures of the body are called *chakras* (CHOCK-ruz). All forms of non-Westernized medicine, Ayurvedic medicine, traditional Chinese medicine, homeopathy, and indigenous cultures around the world acknowledge that a vital life-force energy creates and sustains physical life. It is called by different names, a few of which are *prana* (subtle life-force energy), *chi*, or *mana*. No matter the name, they all point to the same knowledge: that there is an invisible force that ebbs and flows within all living things and is the animating force of creation, sustenance, and destruction.

Ayurvedic medicine specifies 350 chakras and 72,000 nadis through which prana flows in both the energetic field and physical body. For the purposes of this book, however, I will focus on the seven primary chakras—their locations, physiological associations, and examples from my clients that demonstrate the application of the chakra model to everyday situations.

Each of the primary chakras has a specific color and level of consciousness associated with it. Keep in mind that what I am describing is only a model, and you as an individual need not necessarily follow it exactly.

As you work with your chakras and experience them, you may see, feel, hear, or know a color or a certain thought form of consciousness moving through your body; and what you experience may vary from the standard associations that I will explain. But as I've suggested, such differences are perfectly all right. There is no right or wrong; there is only direction. Simply be an observer and allow it all to happen. These variations result from the chakras being closely interconnected; they reflect your common issues, energies, and behavior. Your body and its energetic system are unique.

When I look at people, I see myriad colors—and you likely will too as you develop your intuitive sense—emanating from their physical bodies, swirling and dancing in a kaleidoscopic manner. These colors can accurately reflect all a person's life experiences, the body's current and past physical structure, behaviors, emotions, and present and potential levels of consciousness.

The seven primary colors of the chakras resemble the colors of a rainbow. The first chakra is red; the second chakra, orange; the third chakra, yellow; the fourth chakra, green; the fifth chakra, sky blue; the sixth chakra, indigo; the seventh chakra, violet. While this is the foundational premise of the colors associated with each specific chakra, other colors can move in and around these colored centers. These variations of color can indicate health, illness, emotional attachments, and a host of other issues. Later in this chapter I will introduce an exercise that incorporates all the colors of the chakras so that you can begin to gain a personal experience and understanding of your own chakra system.

On a physical level, the chakras have the important role of maintaining balance in the body. Energy medicine and its work are based on this role. The chakras effect their role through the endocrine and neurological systems. When your body receives an energetic impact from someone or something, the neurological system is stimulated. The neurological system of the body is the closest to the energetic system in that both are in part electrically based. Neurological impulses subsequently stimulate the endocrine system. The endocrine system (with its ductless glands) and the neurological system are the physical, internal directors maintaining control and balance in your body. These two self-regulating systems continually align and realign the body and mind as they respond to energetic impacts.

As the neurological and endocrine systems work to maintain balance, hormones sometimes flood the bloodstream. Science has shown that hormones affect mood, behavior, motivation, and even physical appearance. They also affect such bodily functions as respiration and digestion. Hormonal secretions can even alter intellectual clarity. It is therefore vital for your physical and emotional wellness that you understand the hormones' effects on your energetic system and their manifestations in your physical condition and health.

Each chakra has the same atomic structure as your physical body—the same atomic structure, in fact, upon which all life is built. Its form is directed into the body's spinal column, hence its direct effect on the neurological and all other systems of the body. Chakras are conical in shape. As I perceive them, a lens-like structure connects the physical spine and the nonphysical chakra. The energetic structure and density of this lens lie somewhere between physical and nonphysical form—similar to the way an element exists between a solid and gaseous state. Your intuition is a device through which you will be able to detect this in-between aspect of your energetic system; consequently, it is imperative that you develop a heightened state of awareness.

This lens-like structure acts as both a conduit and an interpreter. It conducts energetic stimuli from their external source to one or more chakras. From there, the stimuli penetrate more deeply into the denser spinal column and neurological system. The direction of this spread of energy is determined by the emotional components and intentions encoded in the stimulus. Feeling butterflies in your stomach is an example of one response to a stimulus. Obviously, though, there are many types of impacts and corresponding responses to these stimuli in your spirit, body, and mind. I will discuss these in the next chapter.

As you read this book and become acquainted with your own energy system through experiential exercises, you will learn to see, feel, hear, smell, and/or know how to open, balance, and cleanse your personal energy system. Since the chakras are subtle constructs of energy, they have less mass than the physical body and therefore cannot be seen by the physical eye. Also, chakras two through six extend from both the front of the body and the back, while the first and seventh chakras extend downward and upward respectively. Training and practice in developing your intuition will allow you to experience your chakras. The methods by which you will experience your energetic system have been time-tested in the courses I have taught since 1990, as well as by a lifetime of my own experiences. However, these experiences go far beyond you and me; they are documented in most classical texts on spirituality and spiritual practices such as the Hindu, Pali, and Buddhist sutras and Chinese Taoism.

The First Chakra

Location: *Tailbone*
Color: *Red*
Primary Consciousness: *Survival*

Survival and safety are the structural roots of this chakra. The earth, family, body, and other structural aspects of life are all part of the first chakra; the key is that they are all associated with the survival level of consciousness to which we are attached. The body's immune system is associated with the first chakra's survival instincts, as well as the third chakra, which I will discuss shortly.

"Tribal" is a word often associated with this chakra. Carolyn Myss coined the term. Thanks to her amazing intuitive skill and popularity, the brand has become popularized among Westerners. Tribal mentality naturally comes into play within the context of survival; the family or larger culture—the tribe—creates the structures in which we survive in the world. But it is just one aspect of the first chakra. The true meanings of the first chakra are survival, safety, and structure.

This chakra is the basic consciousness upon which all other chakras are built. Consequently, releasing unhealthy attachments to societal conditions regarding survival is essential for achieving higher levels of consciousness and truly feeling the interconnectedness between your being and God and all other beings.

In addition to the primal force of procreation driving us to survive as a species, we may attach a variety of culturally based beliefs to the notion of survival. Insecurities are born in the first chakra, although they might be connected to other chakras. You may, for example, feel a strong need to conform to every whim of society in order to survive or to feel safe or included. Conversely, you might feel a need to be as far removed from societal pressures as possible for your survival. Or, like many, you may be attached to money, having a mate, or being close to family. You might find that you are attached to living in a certain region of the world or in a particular environment. Any demonstration of emotional, behavioral, or language (verbal or nonverbal) patterns related to survival issues stems from first-chakra consciousness and energy.

Physiologically, the first chakra influences the immune system, legs, tailbone, colon, prostate, perineum, and any other tissue or structure in that section of the body. As is widely known, sometimes the colon quickly empties its contents in instances of extreme fear. This is a physiological response to a perceived threat to survival, a first-chakra issue. The external threat or challenge to survival stimulates the first chakra, which in turn affects the neurological system and, finally, the behavior of the colon.

First-chakra consciousness is body-level consciousness. The first chakra is strongly attached to your physical world. The fears, worries, and concerns residing in you related to this chakra will dictate, to a large degree, the level of risk you are willing to take in your life. Working with the various exercises in this book, such as Running the Rainbow, you will become skilled at intuitively examining and sensing your chakras. When you observe the energies that exist at the first-chakra level of perception, your attachments to other people, places, or things will be revealed. It is thus an important area of consciousness and energy to look at within yourself. As with all the other chakra centers, hidden truths will arise. But if they are acknowledged and released by doing the exercises in this book, you will be set free, detached from anything that does not serve your consciousness, energy, body, or way of life.

Georgia, a beautiful and talented woman, came to see me due to severe anxiety. Under the guidance of a doctor, she was taking some medications to relieve her anxiety and help her sleep at night. In discussing her history, she described her unsettling family situation when she was growing up; her first chakra was clearly lighting up as a major point of energetic congestion. To me, it looked like the area's energy was more animated than the surrounding energy. Its textures, temperature, and colors could change and become more fluid, grainy, or dense.

Georgia was holding emotional pain; she was fearful. We talked at length, and I reported to her what her body was telling me: She had fears about abandonment, not expressing herself, and moving forward with her talents. Georgia had been trained as an operatic singer, and when she spoke of her voice and her singing, her body and facial features lit up so beautifully. I sensed in her the strong desire to be able to sing once more.

In talking about the fears that had been so prevalent in her life, Georgia mentioned losing her tailbone in an accident. Obviously the loss of this physiological component of the survival-related chakra had had a profound effect on her. There was a connection, in Georgia's case, between the missing tailbone, the damage to the first chakra, the instability of her childhood, and the anxiety building toward her present emotional state. Fortunately, even though she could not replace the tailbone, she could compensate with a concentrated focus of energy in that area to bring about healing and restore balance. In energy medicine it is believed that where you put your mind's attention, energy will follow; in doing so, it can transform the energetic dynamics of that area of the body. If you alter the energy, you alter the body's chemistry. For Georgia, the healing and restoration of balance there would extend to include the mental, emotional, and physical struggles she was also facing.

The Second Chakra

Location: *Abdominal area*
Color: *Orange*
Primary Consciousness: *Sexual, creative energy*

Everything we manifest in our three-dimensional reality is born from second-chakra energy—whether it is the birth of a baby, an idea, a career path, our income, friendship, partnership, or another type of relationship to the world in and around us.

Physiologically, second-chakra energy governs the reproductive organs, the pelvic structures (both muscular and skeletal), and all other tissues in that area of the body. The endocrine systems are influenced by the second chakra, particularly reproductive and various hormonal functions as well as certain digestive processes. Many disorders and diseases, both physical and emotional, arise from conflicted, dysfunctional perceptions about how to nurture second-chakra creative sexual energy and consciousness.

In my day-to-day practice, I frequently see abuse of second-chakra energy. Not limited to a specific culture, this abuse is evident in all peoples and places throughout the world. Giving away second-chakra energy, or using it to manipulate others, leads to serious imbalances. Such imbalances can include addictive and rebellious behaviors and dysfunctional sexual attitudes and behaviors in both men and women. The constant pressure in the workplace to perform and push one's creative limits can drain away this vital energy. Dissatisfaction with work, career, or colleagues only exacerbates this tendency. Certain cultural and religious attitudes toward men's and women's sexuality represent abuse of this creative energy—in some instances, severe abuse in the form of physical mutilation.

In my healing facilitation work, I see so many parts of the body thrown out of whack because of the stress of misused energy, especially that of the second chakra. A simple example: If you have chronic lower back pain, look at whether you are always using your creative energy in a forceful manner. Do you often feel that you have to over-achieve, fix everybody, or make it your responsibility to create the perfect home, office, child, or project? Certainly, lower back pain can be the result of poor physical posture, but also consider your energetic and emotional posture behind the scenes. Be mindful of how your use of your body's energy is connected to your emotions, behaviors, and perceptions.

Applying willpower to force a particular type of energy affects the backs of the chakras. In the previous examples, forcing your creative energy places undue stress on the back of the second chakra. Anytime you try to push through things that are not flowing well, using your will instead of letting your energy flow naturally, you place stress on the back of the chakra. In the case of the second chakra, forcing your creative, sexual energy can throw your lower lumbar or sacral area out, and if you continue forcing this energy it can affect the organs in the lower abdominal region. Take a moment and think about how you use your will and where in your body it expresses occasional or chronic pain. You don't need to immediately act on the wisdom you gain; let your body absorb it.

I have found that reproductive system diseases in both men and women are usually filled with the emotions of sadness, remorse, revenge, hatred, and exhaustion related to the misuse of second-chakra energy. I have seen too many reproductive systems turned upside down, energetically speaking. Ovaries, uteruses, and their surrounding tissues are full of cysts, fibroids, and cancers that result from women constantly giving away their second-chakra energy.

To give you an idea of how powerful second chakra-related perceptions and behaviors can be, I will share my client Sheila's story. Sheila came to my office after having tried unsuccessfully to become pregnant with the aid of expensive fertility drugs and procedures. She came with the hope of finding out if anything was blocking her emotionally or energetically.

The first picture I saw in my mind's eye was Sheila at the age of seven or so. She was standing with her arms folded across her chest in defiance. She was angry with her mother; the emotional energy of her anger was attached to her mother's energy. In addition, her uterus had taken on the same posture energetically. I saw that it had turned itself around and wouldn't face her mother; it had turned away from the issues during this time in Sheila's childhood. Furthermore, within her electromagnetic field I saw a colorful mass of light. The energetic mass was that of her unborn child's soul. It was floating outside her physical body in the auric field, waiting for Sheila to clear the issues around her mother so it could come into her body and into her life; Sheila, her husband, and their unborn child had a promise to fulfill. I shared with Sheila what I was seeing and sensing, and then I applied healing energy to this specific area and other related areas of her body. She left my office soon after, and several weeks later I got a call from her saying she was pregnant. Seven years later I spoke with her again.

She had obviously done more work on her own because, over the years, she and her husband had celebrated the births of several more happy, healthy children.

The Third Chakra

Location: *Solar plexus or stomach area*
Color: *Yellow*
Primary Consciousness: *Personal power and will*

The third chakra governs the stomach, liver, gall bladder, pancreas, kidneys, adrenal glands, and other organs, tissues, muscles, and skeletal structures in the midsection of the body. The will that is related to third-chakra energy and consciousness is different from the willfulness associated with the backs of the chakras. It is the willpower that drives a person's self-concept. It relates to self-esteem, self-worth, self-confidence, and feelings of empowerment. Of significance, powerful lymph glands reside in the third chakra region; in fact, this chakra's cone-like structure runs right through the part of the body known as gut-associated lymphatic tissue (GALT).

As Elizabeth Lipski, Ph.D., CCN, notes in her book *Digestive Wellness*, "Seventy percent of your body's immune system is located either in or near the digestive tract." In addition, it is well documented in Western medicine that the GALT is where 95 percent of the body's serotonin is produced. Consequently, negative energy impacts on this chakra region can compromise the lymphatic and immune systems, which can subsequently engage the first chakra's survival energies. You might recall becoming ill after getting fired, being rejected by a partner, or going through any other situation that offended your self-worth, self-esteem, or sense of empowerment. Perhaps you even felt the power drain out of your body; that is an example of a first- and third-chakra depletion. When there is nothing, nothing is left to give.

Gloria called me when she found out that she had pancreatic cancer. I worked with her while she was in the hospital. The cancer was
aggressive, and it was clear to me that she had a fight on her hands.
Her loved ones and I conversed out in the hallway, and one of the
things they shared with me was that Gloria had always been afraid of
dogs. It so happened that while she was in the hospital, a seeing eye
dog poked its head into her room. Gloria was terrified, especially
when the German shepherd jumped up on her bed. But according to
her family and friends, the dog was surprisingly loving and gentle with
Gloria—it was like an angel in disguise.

After a few minutes, Gloria calmed down as she realized the dog's
intrusion was a gift that would allow her to finally rid herself of her
fear. They cuddled for quite some time. The experience called on
Gloria to maneuver through her labyrinth of fear. She later died from
the cancer; nonetheless, her ability to face her fear allowed her to
gain some wisdom and understanding about her life and its journey.
Like Gloria, no matter where you are, no matter what your circumstances, sooner or later you will be invited to face your fears and
reclaim your power.

The Fourth Chakra

Location: *Center of the thoracic region*
Color: *Green*
Primary Consciousness: *Unconditional love*

Known as the heart chakra, this chakra's energy is unlike the more
one-dimensional energy of sexual or romantic love. It is unconditional
love that carries the potential for the divine romance between God
and all of creation to occur within each of us.

Physiologically, this chakra governs the lungs, ribs, thymus gland,
and heart, as well as all the other muscles, tissues, and skeletal struc-

tures in the thorax area. I have always found it fascinating that I usually sense whether, how, and how long a person wants to live on this planet by tuning into or placing my hand on his chest. Pictures flow through my mind's eye as to the ease with which he is living his life. Both the difficulties and joys of how it has unfolded, and whether it has unfolded according to his heart's desire, are indicated in this region of the body. Next time you are confused about which direction to take in your life, simply breathe in and out slowly and deeply into the heart chakra region. Place a hand over your chest and listen; feel, see, and sense the direction that is beckoning you with your inner vision.

The heart chakra is also the bridge that links the energy of the lower three chakras and the upper three chakras. The heart chakra is the place where all your chakras' voices can be heard. Take the time to listen to the voices at this chakra; doing so will undoubtedly change your life.

Julia had recently retired when she came to see me. All her life she had given to others—her family, church, schools, businesses, and the community. When she retired from her life's work, which she had dearly loved, her life slowed down enough for her body to relay some important messages to her. Within eighteen months of her retirement, Julia had gone through breast cancer, a mastectomy, and triple bypass heart surgery, and her thyroid had atrophied, nearly killing her. Her body, through her heart chakra, was screaming at her to love herself as much as she had loved and cared for others. It was a powerful, poignant time in her life. Through these health challenges Julia learned balance. She still gave of herself to others, just not all of herself. Eighteen years have passed since then. She is now eighty-three years old and lives a full and engaging life.

Loving and giving to yourself as joyously as to others helps you avoid the resentments that can build up over time if you negate your own desires in favor of others'. In order to give to others, it's necessary to give yourself the things you need. Accomplishing this is a challenge for many women. It is also a challenge for those who don the hat of healer. But it is a lesson that will be learned, one way or another, sooner or later, and so it will be easier if you start listening to the whispers of your body and heart before they become screams.

Unconditional love, spiritual love, divine love, the sustaining love for a partner, child, or parent are all aspects of the relational love brought forth, nurtured, stroked, and sometimes dashed through this energy center. As a human being who has walked on this planet for more than a few years, you have felt both the explosive exhilaration and crushing suppression of heart-chakra energy. Finding and giving love are deeply characteristic aspects of our innate nature as human beings.

Loving God, yourself, and others in an honoring and compassionate way will open your heart center, allowing you to experience amazing levels of bliss, compassion, and satisfaction in life.

The Fifth Chakra

Location: *Throat*
Color: *Sky blue*
Primary Consciousness: *Communication, divine communication, and truthfulness*

The main lesson in connection with this chakra is communicating the truth to yourself and to others.

Physiologically, the throat chakra relates to the thyroid, parathyroid, esophagus, larynx, pharynx, nose, and sinuses. The mouth, teeth, salivary glands, and upper section of the gastrointestinal tract are also governed by the fifth chakra.

Cynthia learned in a directly personal manner the power contained in fifth-chakra consciousness. Years before I met her, she and her husband decided to purchase a business together in her hometown. Her husband quit his job, one that he had been unhappy with, and Cynthia abandoned her pursuit of a college degree. The couple put their house on the market, pulled their children out of school, and relocated.

During their first eight months, the business did very well; the community gave its support and praise, and the financial picture looked good. However, after the summer season had ended, Cynthia's husband decided he wasn't happy and wanted to move back where they'd been living. After much deliberation, Cynthia reluctantly agreed. Although she was unhappy about her husband's reversal, she didn't express her true feelings. She was afraid to because whenever she attempted speak up, her words were often met with an angry and hateful response from her husband. So she remained quiet. Her husband moved on beforehand to start a new job, and Cynthia was left with the tasks of selling the business and a home she and her children dearly loved, pulling the children out of school again, and moving back to rejoin her husband.

Months passed. Cynthia's anger seethed inside because she didn't feel safe enough to express herself; eventually her body reacted. Her throat began to close up, and after consulting with a doctor, she discovered that there was a growth on her thyroid. Not speaking her truth had led her to a physical problem related to the fifth chakra. Her energetic and emotional difficulties stopped the proper flow of life-force energy through her body, which affected her physiology.

Cynthia decided to have surgery to remove the growth and half her thyroid. After the surgery, she became aware of the power of the fifth chakra and has since worked with its energy and consciousness to bring balance to her communication and behavioral patterns. It has been fifteen years since the surgery, and so far she has not had to take any medication due to an imbalance in hormone production in the thyroid. The experience taught Cynthia to speak her truth, to herself and others.

The Sixth Chakra

Location: *Forehead region*
Color: *Indigo*
Primary Consciousness: *Intuition and intellect*

The sixth chakra is also often referred to as the "third eye." Physiologically, it governs the pituitary gland, hypothalamus, eyes, upper sinus tract, and the other matter in that region of the head.

Intuitives love the energy and consciousness of this chakra because it is a place of "empty wisdom," where one can hold a neutral center of attention and intention to go in and accomplish medical intuitive discerning and healing work. It is the safest place from which to do this type of work because it is the place where the energies of neutrality and empty, nonattached wisdom exist.

By focusing your attention on the sixth chakra, you can get into and out of another's energy more safely and perform any corrective measures that might be required; you have a greater chance of remaining unattached to the emotionally based thought forms that are potential causes of another's disorder or disease. This is important because, as you step into another's energy field to do intuitive work, it is essential that you be in a balanced, unbiased state of awareness. Working from the sixth chakra will help ensure this.

If you are not healing others at this time, using the energy of the sixth chakra to pull your intuitive thoughts forward will serve you as well. The sixth chakra exemplifies neutrality. Psychic energy is processed through the third chakra and carries with it the risk of applying personal experiences and bias along with intuitive information. Holding a sixth-chakra focus and feeling the energy up in the forehead, between the eyebrows, indicates that you are directly engaging the sixth chakra. The benefits of this will be accuracy, impartiality, and intuitive precision.

The cyst removed from my brain, which I mentioned in the introduction, was directly aligned with the point at which the back of the sixth chakra extends from the head. The back of the sixth chakra relates to the will of that center—how, when, and where to use sixth-chakra energy and consciousness. When I had my cyst removed, it set off the chain of events of my illness, surgery, blindness, and finally, the marvelous regaining of my inner intuitive sight. And don't worry: There are less extreme ways than brain surgery to open your intuitive center! The sixth chakra is an omnipresent source of extrasensory perception and clairvoyance that is available to everyone.

The Seventh Chakra

Location: *Crown of the head*
Color: *Purple*
Primary Consciousness: *The divine within you and the larger divine universal energy of God, in all its wonderful forms and manifestations*

The well-known chants *om*, *aum*, or *amen*, the universal sounds of God, come from and resonate with the seventh chakra. It is often represented as a thousand-petaled lotus.

Physiologically, the seventh chakra primarily governs the pineal gland. Western science does not fully understand this small gland in the center of the brain; however, some Eastern philosophies refer to it as the seat of the soul. The seventh chakra's energy cannot help but affect the pituitary and hypothalamus as well as the pineal, but it is a secondary influence.

Medical issues related to the seventh chakra are anxiety, nervous system disorders, Parkinson's, Alzheimer's, and most mental illness. Whenever the brain tissue and nervous system are strongly affected, the seventh chakra is involved, as there are separations from one's spiritually divine and physical natures.

A rather fun sensation that you can experience in the seventh chakra is that wonderful tingling sensation at the crown of the head. A student of mine likened it to "feeling bees" at the top of her head. This sensation is a common energetic phenomenon, especially when you are engaged in spiritually based practice. The telltale sensations at the top of the head are often felt when you are deep in prayer or meditation. It is a signal that all is well and that you are connected to God's omnipresence.

Perhaps you can think back to a time when you felt this buzzing at the top of your head; what you were feeling was energetic activity in and around your seventh chakra. Something or someone may have been trying to communicate some information to you energetically. The next time this happens to you, try remaining still and paying attention to any internal guidance or intuitive thoughts you get. You will, in this way, commit to your wisdom.

When the seventh chakra is fully engaged, one has moments of genius. Focus on the top of your head; while in a still and meditative space, you can sense the energy of this center moving. The electric energy shoots across the top of your head in oscillating patterns.

Connecting with the power and consciousness of the seventh chakra can lead you to pure rapture, unity, and bliss. You will feel the purity of your being, for there is no subjective or objective reality: You are truly one with the Source.

Now that you have a clear understanding of your personal energy system, in the next chapter we will look at the many ways in which this system is influenced, how it can affect your physical well-being, and what you can do to heal yourself—body, mind, and spirit.

Recommended Exercises

Running the Rainbow
Dealing with Blockages

5

The Issues Are in the Tissues:
Healing the Body

You Are the Creator of Your Anatomy

As a medical intuitive, I have come to know that we are literally the creators of our anatomy. You construct your body through the innumerable events and encounters with people and other stimuli that enter your life and energetic field over time. Your body, your life, and the emotional and behavioral components with which you manage your world are all interrelated energetic patterns resulting from events that have left their imprints on your personal energy system. It doesn't matter whether the imprinting process is the result of a traumatic experience or a joyful one. It is how you hold onto the situation or memory—emotionally, behaviorally, and especially energetically—that matters. And the way you hold onto something depends on the way in which you perceived what happened to you in the first place.

Your memories of your experiences, the people who raised you, who you went to school with, played with, made love to, married, gave birth to, worked with, and so on, influence how you write your energetic and physical body's story. All these stored memories are actors, in a sense, assisting you in both the writing and presentation of your anatomy. As you move through your life and its myriad experiences, these actors interact with your energy, rehearsing and performing the lessons you are here to learn, as well as those you are here to teach others. You have authored your anatomy based on how you have lived your life up to this point.

It is important to consider whether these influences serve you in the context of your current life or state of being. Take a thoughtful look inside yourself for a moment. From what truths have you been creating your anatomy, and therefore your life? Your own or others'? Do these truths serve you? Do they honor who you are or what you want to become?

Thoughts, emotions, and words have more influence on your body than you might think. In *The Hidden Messages in Water*, Dr. Masaru Emoto demonstrates how words affect the molecular structure of water. According to pictorial documentation of his research, beautiful snowflake-like and crystalline structures occur in water's molecules when words or thoughts of a positive nature are spoken to it: when the water has been exposed to such words (and their respective frequencies) as love, peace, joy, and gratitude. One can project these thoughts with a particular spoken word, a written word, or word groupings such as prayers. You can even place the words on paper and wrap the paper around the water's container to transform the water molecules.

Not surprisingly, the molecules also react to cruel and negative words. Words like hate and kill distort and contort the water molecules so severely that they look like they are on fire, bubbling hot, and deeply irregular. Interestingly enough, when I first saw these pictures, especially the ones resulting from negative thought projections, my first remarks were that these distorted water molecules looked identical to the way in which I saw cells contorted with diseases such as cancer.

Dr. Emoto's research illustrates the power of words, the energy of both spoken and unspoken thought, and the positive or damaging results they can have on water molecules. After reading these brief points from Dr. Emoto's work, I'm certain it has not escaped your attention that our bodies are 70 percent water. It provokes one to think about the effects that words, thoughts, and emotions have on us and on others.

You are indeed the creator of your anatomy. Everything you think, feel, do, and know determines the health and condition of your body, as well as feeding or starving your soul. As a medical intuitive, I have yet to come upon a disorder, dysfunction, or disease in the body that does not have emotional and behavioral components attached to it. The nourishment you have given or allowed yourself to receive, or have lacked, is most definitely evident in the energetic core of a disease.

Energetic Emotional Impact

In my work assisting people, I have been privileged to deal with a wide variety of diseases and disorders: cancer, fibromyalgia, chronic fatigue syndrome, digestive disorders, candida, panic attacks, diabetes, spinal issues, respiratory disorders—the list goes on and on. All the people I have assisted in dealing with these disorders have had a variety of emotions packed inside them at the point of disease, or what I call the point of "emotional/energetic congestion." The evidence of these emotions and their behavior patterns tells both me and the client that she has been either holding or losing her life-force energy in regard to a particular situation, traumatic experience, or person in her life. It is also likely that these issues have been affecting her for some time—in some instances, they have been stuffed down inside her for decades.

To help you understand what is happening when the body holds the energetic imprint of certain experiences or people, let me explain what I call the "energetic emotional impact" theory. Simply stated, this theory is based on the fact that during the early stages of life, prior to achieving certain levels of cognitive maturation, we don't have the ability to understand what happens to us by applying logic to pick a situation apart. The energetic result is that since we don't have these cognitive abilities to figure out traumas, we are left with the only things we have—the emotions and their impact. The intensity of the emotional impact and how the event is perceived control whether any resulting emotional and behavioral patterning will be created. This holding of energy, packed with emotions, results in moving the energy into the physical body on a cellular level. The energetic emotional impact takes up residence in the chakra system.

A trauma can be considered perceptually subjective in nature. Depending on how it's perceived, a trauma can be anything from not having your drawing selected by your fourth-grade teacher to child abuse or the loss of a parent. Certain events when we're young have effects beyond our understanding and control. We simply lack the cognitive means to draw upon. As adults, we can understand why we have been fired or why a marriage hasn't worked. But as children we find it difficult to understand why we feel abandoned, or why we are locked away in a closet or told to go out and cut a switch from a tree so our father can whip us with it. We are left with the emotions associated with these events, and this is the reason people usually have such difficulty healing early childhood issues. Often, when we work on these issues as adults, the emotions pour out like thunderous floodwaters.

To illustrate this, let's look at a typical childhood incident. You fall off your tricycle when you're three years old. A sibling, parent, playmate, or even a stranger tells you, for example, that you're stupid or clumsy for falling off your tricycle. So not only did you scrape your knee and elbow, but your emotional and energetic body was also injured as a result of the hurtful words. The emotional impact—the hurt feelings—thus creates the conditions for the behavioral patterning to begin its existence in a particular chakra.

In this example, you grew up having your feelings hurt when someone directed at you what you perceived to be hateful words. As an adult, you doubt you have the ability to do things well. Or the childhood incident and subsequent experiences made you more determined to try harder when you attempt new things, creating the conditions for becoming an overachiever. The effects depend on your perception of a particular event.

I'd like to share some of my clients' stories to give you a clearer picture of how energetic emotional impacts can play out in your health and wellness.

Samantha

I did an intuitive assessment over the phone with Samantha. She listened as I intuitively dissected one of her ovarian cysts. The energy of this particular cyst was such that I could divide it up into three sections. Each section held energy that appeared to deal with various traumas that had affected her emotionally and behaviorally throughout the years. Each was clearly marked energetically with a specific age indicating at what time in her life the trauma had occurred. I also noticed that relationships had been established with other parts of her physical and energetic anatomy (the chakras), as well as with her spiritual and emotional/behavioral anatomies. In short, all parts of her being had, to different degrees, been affected by these traumas.

The far right section of the particular cyst I was examining held the emotions of anger and frustration. Both of these emotions were associated with her not being able to express her true self from a very early age. This experience had affected not only her second chakra where the cysts were located but also her fifth chakra, the throat. Chronic sore throats, symptomatic of repressed anger, were a constant part of her life. She was taught as a child that it was not okay to express anger, creating an emotional/behavioral pattern that supported the stuffing down of her emotions.

The middle section of the cyst held deep sadness, and it was the basis for her perceived inability to pursue what she really wanted to do. Within her energetic system, this issue corresponded to the age of three years old. I discovered the age association as I looked deep within her personal energy system and saw in my mind's eye a picture of her as a three-year-old being told to hurry up and come along to do something. Also evident in this picture were her feelings of simply wanting to be left alone to play with her toys. She confirmed that what I was seeing made sense, and that she disliked interruptions while engrossed in a task. She added that she didn't allow herself much time, if any, to play and have fun.

The last section of the cyst contained pictures of her not being able to do things right, and of not believing in herself. This corresponded with the energy in her third chakra, which reflected a lack of self-esteem. This energetically charged emotional pattern had produced fear, preventing her from being willing to try new things. But she was tired of missing out on new opportunities. This particular energy, wrapped in these specific emotional reactions, had also affected her solar plexus chakra, resulting in her having to deal with a nervous stomach for many years. Her situation is a clear example of the relationships that are fostered and maintained through the processes of energetic emotional impacts and the effects they can have on physical health.

Barbara

Barbara had been suffering from bouts of asthma for many years and, more recently, frustration over her work in a bureaucratic setting. As she lay on my examination table, I placed my hand on her chest over her thymus gland and asked her why there was such deep sadness and emotional constriction, stemming from around the age of four. I asked, "What have you been disowning about who you are since that time?"

Long-held-back tears began running down her cheeks. She told me that she used to see lights and sparks of color dancing outside her bed-room window at night. She knew that they were guides of some kind, her special guides, trying to relay information to her. She also knew that she knew too much about Spirit, about God, and that the family in which she had been born would not tolerate a young child with so much intuitive, spiritual information. As a result, she shut down. The lights and feelings of interconnection with God left her.

From that time on, she began to make herself into the four-foot, eleven-inch bulldozer she became (my term for her), which helped her manage her life from a point of view that seemed more acceptable but was different from what was true to her intrinsic self. However, by eventually changing how she interacted with her inner self, her family, and the world around her, she began her journey back to herself and her true power. She has since been in the process of rediscovering her incredible intuitive healing abilities and marvelous artistic gifts. Although it took her forty-some years to tell that part of her life's story to someone else, it is a drop in the bucket compared to the time of her soul's existence.

Jennifer

A school bus? Now what does a school bus have to do with this woman's neck and her broken collarbone? I thought to myself as I dug further into the recesses of my intuition. "Now don't think this is too weird," I said to Jennifer, a first-time client, "but did you ride a bus to school around the age of five?" Five came up because I was intuitively seeing that there was a relationship between the school bus, her neck, age five, and a pattern of inhibited communication that had been locked in her energetic, emotional, and behavioral being since that time.

As our session continued, we discovered some interesting things related to the inhibited communication patterns she had been working on, as well as to issues around her broken collarbone. Later that evening, however, Jennifer called me and left a message about what she had discovered. After our session, she had talked to her mother about my comments regarding the school bus and the restricted energy in her neck.

Jennifer said that her mother started laughing when she told her of the school bus popping up in our session. "Don't you remember your first day of school?" her mother asked her. When Jennifer answered that she didn't remember, her mother reminded her that on her first day of school at the age of five she had fallen asleep on the bus and ended up riding past the school drop-off point. It wasn't until the driver came back to the bus at noon that she was startled awake. She missed her entire first day of kindergarten as a result. She didn't consciously remember the experience, but it was there in her body's energetic and emotional memory.

Perceiving Traumas Energetically

Let me explain how I perceive traumas that are energetically lodged in the physical body. Knowing this may help you work more deeply with your own intuitive wellness. When I am in the process of intuitive energetic assessment and looking into a person's energy system, one of the things I see is what I call a "rift," which is caused by a strong energetic emotional impact. As I described in the previous chapter, the chakras are conical in shape and energetically attach to the spinal column at various locations. The narrowest point of the chakra is attached at the spine and then the larger aspect of the chakra's cone moves outward through the body and extends beyond it, on average, six to eight inches. The rift I see appears as a section of a chakra's wall that is out of alignment. There are usually a multitude of rifts in a chakra. All of us have them—they are inescapable—but they are not necessarily bad.

Imagine you are looking at the rings of a tree trunk that reveal the number of years of its growth. Similarly, when I look at a chakra, I see thousands of concentric rings making up the body of the chakra. These rings are all stacked one on top of the other, much like those plastic expandable travel cups you can buy at a drugstore. When a rift occurs in a chakra, it is as if one of the rings has been jerked out of place, causing an expansion in that portion of the chakra wall, which then leads to an energetic swelling in that area. The swelling keeps the rift in this dislodged position and creates a holding area, a memory of the emotional energy that impacted the area and forced it out in the first place.

Furthermore, you create behavior to manage the effects of the impact of energy. If, for example, you were in a severe car accident as a young child, you may not think about it every time you get into the car, but your body and the affected chakras will remind you whenever you get into a traffic situation where you feel a bit more pressure.

When you have an experience in which the energy currents match those of the initial emotional impact, it engages those energetically based emotional and behavioral components in you, thus bringing back the impact memory. So, for example, if something happened when you were young that had a certain emotional, energetic quality and, as you grew up, the same emotional, energetic qualities came at you again, the rift would be reinforced. Your behavioral response to the situation would also be reinforced. By determining the location of the rift (or rifts) relative to the distance from the spinal column, I can gain a better understanding of the relationship between the energy and the emotional impact, as well as the age at which the trauma took place. From this information, I can discover and assess relationships to other chakra components and apply corrective measures.

This ability is within your grasp, too. Whether you have a full-blown disease or are just feeling out of balance, there is a voice encapsulated within your disease, disorder, or misalignment. It is a voice that will direct you and allow you to map out the various impacts and causes of what is happening in your body. It is up to you to intuitively guide your senses and mind inside to where your body's wisdom resides, then listen, pay attention, and act on the information provided.

As you both process and progress, keep in mind that in all instances in life, the power of an impact on any system depends on the energy and intention that are brought to bear, and how both are perceived. So when you become aware of and examine a past issue in your life and its emotional impact, you need to look at the energetic impact itself, the intention of the energy that hit you, and how much power you gave the situation. This is the first set of determinations you need to make when you run across a past event that is still troubling you today.

At the end of this book there are exercises to help you access the voice of your inner wisdom. Before you look through them, I'd like to discuss further factors that can influence your personal energy system.

Locating Disharmony Within Your Body

Illness can be an effective way for our souls to get our attention. Taking a deeper look into the components of illness can assist us in unlocking the mystery of how our thoughts, emotions, and behaviors may have created disharmony in us. Understanding what has brought us to a certain place enables us to better handle the situation and find solutions more effectively. Awareness is essential.

One of the many natural laws that govern the universe is that all structures are made of energy and have mass. In addition, the energy that constitutes a particular mass has a vibrational rate that supports, and therefore identifies, that mass. Thus, vibrational rates vary from one mass to another. A simple example taken from the earth's body is that the molecular structure of a rock vibrates at a different rate from that of water. On the level of your body, your bones' molecular structure vibrates differently from that of your blood.

With this in mind, if there is, say, a misalignment in your body's system, a vibration will arise that is not within its normal structural and energetic vibratory range. That discordant energy's vibration announces that something is wrong, out of harmony. Using this principle I can discern when a part of the body is out of harmony with its surrounding tissues or structures—I can see, feel, hear, or know the disharmony in the body's vibrations. And so can you. Be mindful that, at times, we become content with this unhealthy vibration. We ignore the imbalance and begin to think that it is normal. We settle into a state of complacency or victimization. Consequently, we push harder to make things work in our lives, discount our bodies, and renounce our heart's desires. We lose the connection to our natural flow.

Here's a story illustrating this point. While my sister Christine and I were traveling in northern Arizona, we checked into a hotel near the Petrified Forest. The young man who assisted us was of Native American descent. We enjoyed a brief but interesting discussion about spirituality and universal oneness. Later that evening, Christine went to get a soda. Her attempts at the machine were unsuccessful, however; the machine would not accept one of her dimes no matter what she did. The young man who had helped us check in walked over to see if he could be of any assistance. Christine gave him the dime, and he placed it in the slot only to have the same result. The dime slid down inside the belly of the machine and plopped out into the coin return. After a few attempts, he calmly picked up the dime, handed it back to my sister, and concluded, "This dime is not in harmony with the machine." He smiled and walked away.

Imagine the machine is your body, your energy, or your life. The dime can be anything or anyone who comes into your existence and slides right through, offering you no return for your efforts or wishes, and possibly causing your body's energetic vibrational rate to be out of harmony. Whatever or whomever your dime represents, it is important for you to see why your attempt to put it into your body is not working; it is important to know why it is not in harmony with what you need or desire.

Your soul's health is expressed through the various systems and places in your physical body. By listening deeply to your intuition, you can locate the source of your disharmony. Any pain in your body is a signal from your soul. The pain points to a disorder. In effect, your body is the mouthpiece through which the soul speaks.

There may be cries sounding deep within you, yet you might not hear them or know what they are about. At times these soul-level pleas end up being pushed down further inside where you are even less likely to hear them. Over time, you move so far away from your inner source that your soul becomes a total stranger to you. When this occurs, energy, thoughts, and emotions begin to grate against the core of your being, creating what I call psychophysical dissonance and energetic disharmonies. These conditions slowly gnaw away at the physical body. As I have seen over and over again, we will become ill, sometimes deathly ill, if we don't listen to and act on our soul's voice and its directives.

I received a call one day from a woman named Wendy who wanted to make an appointment for an intuitive reading with me. She was crying and obviously distraught. She recounted how she had been through a cavalcade of physicians over the past few years—allopathic, naturopathic, and homeopathic. Some had recommended taking certain herbal formulas and promised that if she did so she would be well in a matter of weeks. Others had suggested a blood test or CAT scan. She went back and forth with the more alternative-oriented doctors, as she was wary of invasive tests. However, Wendy's condition was worsening, and she didn't know what to do.

As we talked, I shared with her my point of view: Sometimes when you are ill, herbs can be the perfect remedy; other times you may need castor oil packs, meditation, or traditional methods of diagnosis and sometimes even surgery. I asked her what her body had to say about what she should do. Wendy didn't know, she admitted; she had never asked. I suggested that she ask and see what wisdom her body had to share with her.

Although I didn't do a formal reading while we were on the phone, I encouraged her to listen to her body's wisdom and advocated that she seek out a traditional physician. I also suggested she talk to her stomach area in particular. The cells in her digestive tract appeared swollen and inflamed. There was severe energetic congestion there, holding fear and anger. Wendy called me back a week later, and to my surprise, her voice was full of joy and elation. She told me that when she talked to her body and listened to it, it told her to get the CAT scan, along with other, more traditional tests. And she did just that. It may seem odd that Wendy's voice was filled with joy when in fact the test results showed she was heading into the advanced stages of stomach cancer and had only a 30 percent chance of survival. But the beginning of her healing was in the knowing, and in the new connection she had made with her body and the emotions it held.

Illnesses are signals from your soul, inviting you to go deep within yourself, to start listening to the real source of your being. Your soul's voice is accessible intuitively, and that is why it is so important that you develop this type of intuitive connection to your inner self. When you honor your intuition, it will be easier for you to hear your soul's cry for help and make the adjustments needed to put you in accord with your inner truths.

Our Intrinsic Energy Pattern

A key way to avoid energetic disharmonies is to get back to your intrinsic energy pattern. Each of us is born with an energetic pattern that is a clear reflection of our soul's pure nature. However, as we move through our lives absorbing one experience after another, we tend to correct, or alter, this intrinsic pattern. We form a new one that we hope will allow us to manage our lives based on the information and experiences we receive from such external sources of authority as our families and the various cultural institutions—religious, educational, governmental, and economic—around us. The common responses of conformity and appeasement and their attendant behaviors, along with the suppression of our emotions, cause untold emotional and health problems.

Your own truths are deeply encoded inside your intrinsic energy pattern. They are, nonetheless, accessible. The natural wondrousness of who you are, along with all the talents and gifts you have brought into this lifetime, are contained there. The talents and gifts you possess are expressed through your heart.

When I was in the depths of my near-death experience and on the other side, my communication with those who were there with me was from heart to heart. There were no vocal interactions as we usually think of them. Everything was expressed from one soul to another through the heart center. And you came into this world with the same level of openness in your heart center. Children's openness and heartfelt expressiveness toward the world demonstrate this.

Somewhere along life's route, however, this openheartedness becomes suppressed. When for whatever reason this closing off takes place, the connection with your intrinsic energy pattern, which speaks through your heart center, gradually becomes lost. And as a result of this loss, you can lose sight of your innate talents and gifts. Unfortunately, I often witness this type of disconnection when I work with people in the office or on the phone. Even if they are usually joyful and pleasant people, helpful and kind, on the deeper, private levels, their heart centers have been hurt along the way and closed down to varying degrees as a means of protection.

Over and over, I have worked with closed-down chakras and the health problems that result. I have often seen prostate and colon disorders (hemorrhoids, too) that are the result of early childhood imprinting by parents still dealing with memories of the Great Depression. Money is generally a second-chakra issue, but for many people money is placed in a survival context, turning it into a first-chakra issue. This can therefore affect the first and second chakras and their corresponding anatomical components. Many people build their whole lives on this fear of lack. A life built on any fear is simply not a good idea. I have seen clients who were very successful in life and in business but who nevertheless, based on their early programming, squeezed the life-force energy out of their first and second chakras, in effect shutting them down and causing these types of illnesses.

In female clients, I have seen many diseased ovaries, breast cancer cases, and dysfunctional thyroids because of distorted internal pictures related to body size, sexual issues, creativity, abuse, and the inability to express their true selves. All these concepts and experiences can result in shutting down the respective chakras. Holding in deep hurt and disappointment damages the heart chakra, often leading to breast cancer and heart disease.

These are examples of how I see energy being held in the body as a result of something having happened that closes our innate openheartedness. This closure usually originates in a self-created myth that it is no longer safe to be who you intrinsically are. When you close down the heart chakra, or any other chakra of your body's energetic system, it affects your intrinsic energy pattern—away from a primarily heart-centered openness to a new, distorted energetic pattern. This new pattern offers a way to manage your life but, disconnected from this deeper aspect, it masks your talents and weakens your passion to express them. Eventually, you get used to this dullness and it becomes a part of how you are in the world. You might tell yourself this new way is tolerable, but I assure you that it is not. It is critical that we all rewire ourselves and go back to our intrinsic energy patterns, and thus live true to ourselves once again.

Paul, for example, had been working in the technology field for several years. He faced a long commute each day, only to sit in an office that he hated. He had managed to create a schedule in which he worked one day of the week at home on the computer, but there was still a great deal of pain and suffering in his heart and in his body. As a result of tolerating his situation and misdirecting his energy as he did, he had lost his vitality and passion for life. He revealed to me that what he really wanted to do was write and make audiotapes of children's stories from a spiritual perspective.

During our session together, it became clear that Paul had re-formed himself according to a socially constructed reality and was managing his life in a way that he thought would make it a little better. He had completely rewired himself and his energetic system to fit a mold that somebody else—his father—had made for him. This is not to place blame on his father, since we all have a soul-level role in every interaction we encounter. Paul's issue was that his physical and energetic power was weakening quickly and he needed to get his vitality, passion, and energetic system back into alignment; that meant he needed to do some inner work.

Before describing Paul's intrinsic energy pattern, I first want to make a comment about the workings of these patterns in general. We all have unique ways in which we access, process, and display our energy. We use the seven primary chakras to form our intrinsic pattern. The chakras light up, in a manner of speaking, in different ways and in a different order based on who a person is on an intrinsic, soul level. When I see the first chakra light up I know that it is the predominant chakra of a person's system, the core of who he is. Everything builds from there. It holds his archetypal personality traits, spiritual lessons, and gifts. The order of lighting up that follows indicates not only the positive side of his personality and life path, but the shadow side as well. It reflects the aspects of his personality that drive his life's lessons—good or bad.

Given that, Paul's intrinsic pattern was as follows. The energy came into his body first through his sixth chakra, the intuitive center (Paul is extremely intuitive, but, at the time of the reading, he didn't know how to access or use his intuitiveness to his benefit). Next—but virtually simultaneously—his intuitive center's energy flowed down to his second chakra, his creative energy center located in the lower abdomen. That accumulated energy then dropped down even further to his tailbone, the first chakra. This energy then sat in the first chakra, lighting it up, and made him feel comfortable and safe (the first chakra, as you might recall, is primarily about survival and safety).

After fueling the first chakra, the energy moved up his body's energy channels and into his heart chakra. At this point, it was as if his energy checked in with the writings of his soul to make sure he was in alignment. Then the energy would spread a great deal of joy throughout his entire body. The core of his energy then moved from the heart chakra up into the throat chakra, where the energy of what he was working on could be expressed, to others and himself. Finally, after expressing this intuitively based creative and secure heart energy, it all sank into his power center (the third chakra), where his self-esteem was nurtured and empowered. This gave him a strong sense of self-confidence. His seventh-chakra energy was more like a frame for his entire body as it wrapped all around him, feeding him from every angle.

Paul is a spiritually directed person, as demonstrated by the above description of his intrinsic pattern, but he had been running his life as far away as he could get from this energy pattern. If you recall, his sixth chakra (his intuitive center) was the center that naturally led his energetic parade and was his most natural and appropriate perspective on the world, while his third (heart) chakra was basically the last in line. During our session, however, I discovered that he has been running his life with his third chakra leading the way. He was thus out of balance; his "life's dime" was not in harmony. As a result, his body's health and his energy level had been slowly fading for years.

Correct Imbalances by Listening to Your Soul's Voice

As Paul's story demonstrates, going against innate truths and ignoring our soul's voice, a voice that directs us toward our gifts and talents, is often the root of the manifestation of disorders and diseases. Instead of answering the call to make a living at what we love, we go into careers that are expected of us or what our families want us to do. It is unhealthy to do something for a living that you are not intrinsically suited for. You must figure out who you are and then, if you want to, do who you are for a living. In this way, you will live a much more rewarding, consciously soulful life. Americans have more heart attacks at 9:00 Monday mornings than any other group of people on this planet. It appears that people have totally disconnected from their heart's desires and their intrinsic energy patterns, becoming and doing what they are not.

Life is not easy at times and it can be challenging to live your life with the outer world pressing against you. In order to find some inner peace and healing, we need to find the balance between two opposing poles. One pole is the group mind. At this end, the individual and individuality are totally lost in a sea of group consciousness. The other is the individual mind maintaining a hermit-like existence outside the culture's precepts, morals, and values.

We need be able to comply to some degree with our culture's norms and mores in order to avoid chaos. On the other hand, we need to honor and be honored for who we are as individuals. To that end, it is imperative that we know and understand what our inner truths are and how we can maintain our personal, soul-based sense of integrity in the context of the surrounding culture. Balance between internal and external authority is key.

Find balance between the two by knowing what your inner truths are. The surrounding culture and its various institutions have done their job of bringing you up as a model citizen (whether you agree with the ideal or not). However, what you have been taught is true may differ, slightly or a lot, from the deeper internal truths of your soul. It is important to look deeply into what you believe about yourself, your world, and the way you move through your world, because the way you move through it—energetically, emotionally, spiritually, and physically—actually creates every part of your body's cellular structure.

Decoding Your Inner Graffiti

To discover your innate truths, you have to get in there and look through the patterns of your life and see where you are not honoring your soul's truth. Be your own archaeologist and dig up your hidden treasures. You need to look at how you may have rewired yourself and your energy to please, appease, and placate others. An important first step in discovering these things is decoding your inner graffiti.

By inner graffiti, I'm referring to the socially constructed inner writings that have been painted on your soul's walls, so to speak—the internalized vocal patterns that repeat themselves over and over in your mind. We all have them; you cannot live in a culture and not have them. You will recognize, if you haven't already, that your graffiti is constantly bouncing off the walls of your mind. In order to cut through it, you've got to practice stilling your mind chatter. Once you gain some of this stillness, you will naturally begin to see that your graffiti-like chatter is not inherently yours; rather, you've been holding it for someone else. And you don't need to hold onto it any longer. You can move it out of your mind, body, and energy patterning. Quieting the mind is the beginning of this process and discernment will follow, allowing you to wipe the graffiti from your soul's walls.

In the yoga posture tree pose (*vrikshasana* in Sanskrit) one stands on one foot with the other placed either at the inside of the opposite knee or high up on the inside of the opposite thigh. If you attempt this posture with your inner graffiti flying hither and yon, your balance will be affected and the tree (you) will wobble or fall. A still mind is a still body, and on the contrary, a chattering, graffiti-filled mind will throw you off and make it difficult for you to see the foreign scrawl on the walls of your soul.

At first it may be a challenge to distinguish your soul's voice from your inner graffiti, which has various tones and levels of intensity. These voices are constantly vying for your attention, whispering or shouting, hoping you will listen to them and do what they say. Although some of these voices are indeed from your soul and various parts of your physical body, offering you wisdom and instruction as to what to feed your body and how to move it, others beckon you, for example, to eat things that don't serve your body's health. You can often identify inner graffiti as random programmed thoughts repeating like a broken record. These repetitive voices form a chant of sorts and are the ones with the most power to lead you astray from your soul's voice.

If the interference of voices grows, you will most likely begin to acquire excesses in your life. These excesses may manifest as added stress, added weight, or too many people telling you to do this or that. Or you may just start collecting objects to feed your starving soul. To get rid of the excess in your life, you need to clear the mud from your mind, listen to your body's pleas, and take a close look at the interior walls of your soul where the cumulative graffiti of your life has been scrawled.

Developing a practice of meditation will help you accomplish this. Turning your attention inward, toward the inner peace of the soul and the feeling of bliss you experience as you connect deep within your heart chakra, will help you recognize and resist your chattering mind. Take time during your day to go into this peaceful inner sanctuary; if you desire to clean up your outer world, you must take the time to tidy up what is inside you.

Listening to your body is another simple but powerful method to get in touch with your soul's voice. Your soul will speak to you through the various organs and components of your physical body. Listen to your body and it will tell you what you need to do for yourself. The key is listening to and then trusting the information that comes through. To build this trust, you need to practice discerning, listening to, and trusting the voice of your soul.

Decoding your inner graffiti also involves getting down to your intrinsic energetic self. Like any other spiritual quest, this does not necessarily consist of sudden, miraculous events (although the occasional epiphany is possible). You needn't worry about diving in and doing this deep kind of work and expect to undergo "the big change." For the most part, deep soul changes are the result of commitment to the search and a gradual process of shifts in consciousness.

I often refer to the decoding process using the analogy of concrete. Concrete consists of hundreds and hundreds of pieces of aggregate. In the sand alone, there are billions of individual pieces constituting the whole. Water is also part of the mixture. All these components, when mixed together, bind to create what seems to be a hard reality.

Likewise, your spirit, mind, body, and energetic system have been bound together by the pieces of aggregate of your habitual behaviors, emotions, and instinctual pressures. Decoding your inner graffiti is taking a symbolic sledgehammer and lovingly dismantling the concretized pieces of your life so you can get to your core.

Your inner graffiti interferes with your ability to access your deepest soul self. Understanding the chakras' construction and finding the rifts in the system is one of the ways you can start decoding your inner graffiti. Unraveling the behavioral, emotional, and energetic patterns you have created in your life is a primary step toward creating balance and harmony; it allows you to tap into your deeply held innate wisdom. As your deep sources of wisdom bubble to the surface, healing and growth will begin to occur—physically, energetically, emotionally, and spiritually.

The power needed for you to grasp your inner graffiti and change things in your life exists within you; it can be called upon by your will and with some applied courage and positive emotions. Sometimes you need to be brave to begin the process of freeing yourself. Be willing to think about being brave. As Maya Angelou said, "It takes courage to have courage." To do this type of deep inner work, it's often helpful to give yourself permission and the space to be where you are. So begin the process gently. You may need to simply be in a place where you are just thinking about acting on your body's wisdom or your soul's voice. That's fine. Remember, you don't have to jump headlong into a situation; just be willing to look at it, and go from there. Any journey begins where you are currently standing.

Changing Your Reality

From physical experiences, you perceive your body as a solid reality. The environment and even the current habits of your reality are perceived by you and supported by the culture as hard reality. However, they have been constructed and are maintained by your mind and set firmly into your body. The mind then keeps you and your body bound to the illusion, which occasionally retards the healing process.

Add to this the fact that as a human being, you also deal with instinctual pressures and universal archetypal forces, and you have quite a tangle to unravel. Instinctual pressures are emotions from past lives that have not been released. They are lodged within, creating habits, feelings, and fears—of fire, falling, water, and so on—that can seem irrational. They can manifest themselves as either dynamic forces or weaknesses that percolate up and gradually find their way into your consciousness and behaviors. Such behaviors combine with cultural constructs to form the superstructure of your life. Of course, you can perceive these behavioral tendencies as either beneficial or not.

You might at times have given up attempting to change your reality because you don't believe you can punch through its hardness. You may believe that the constraints pressing against you are so severe that you cannot be freed from them. You feel out of control and believe that the expressions of your mind, manifested in your body, have taken over; in a word, you feel powerless. But you are not powerless! Your task within any reality you have built is to process and grow on a soul level within that reality. The way to move from one reality, pleasant or horrific, is to learn those soulful lessons and then embrace them.

No matter what you face, you need to understand that the constraining, habit-bound reality marked by frailty, fear, and uncertainty has mental origins that are now locked in your body. But you have the key. You can unlock the door and set yourself free. You are in control of the mental origin of this reality. Certainly it can seem to be a vicious cycle when habit-bound mental tapes replay disaster after disaster in your mind, ultimately affecting your body and environment. However, you must remember that your immortal soul is in control— not your mind, personality, the imprinting you've received, or your enculturation. You are the powerful one who has choreographed the reality in which you exist and move. As an immortal soul in existence since the beginning of time, you have orchestrated your lessons. You can indeed break through seemingly impenetrable realities.

When I was on the road to recovery from the illness that caused my near-death experience, the doctors told me my eyesight would never improve. They also told me I would probably be on medication for the rest of my life. They told me there were lots of things I wouldn't be able to do anymore. In fact, some people around me suggested I apply for Social Security benefits because I would no longer be employable. At the time of my recovery, I had lost my left field of vision in both eyes; I could only see half of whatever I looked at. If I had believed the hard reality that faced me, especially when it came to the issue of my blindness, I would not be where I am today.

I am no longer on any medication, nor did I give up being a productive wage earner for my children and myself. My point is, please don't tell yourself you can't do something because the external reality is too hard for you to break through. You can decode it, learn your soul's lessons from it, then pop that reality bubble, scattering it to the winds.

Create the health and quality of life you desire. You have the God-given power to do so. Believe me, I know about hard realities. I also know about the depth and power of the human spirit. You are in charge of your mind and therefore your reality, inside and out.

Asking your body and then trusting its wisdom can bring you experiences that build belief in your intuitive wisdom. The deepening belief you build through your experiences will in turn enhance and strengthen your discipline and commitment to your growth. Clients with whom I'm working will often say something to the effect that their intuition has been telling them to eat a certain food or perform their practice or live a specific way. Whenever they ask for my opinion, I always offer the same counsel: "Commit to your intuitive wisdom and trust that." I assure them that it's fine if they need to hear their intuition speak to them on a certain issue a few more times. It doesn't matter if you need to hear your inner voice sing out five, fifty, or five hundred more times before you act, as a lesson is contained in that voice each time you hear it. If you choose to listen more quickly, you will get the bigger picture faster and move on without having to experience everything that could potentially be attached to the situation. But don't think there are any shortcuts. You need to listen, examine, and act. You cannot skip these processes to move along your path more swiftly. Your efforts and commitment will move you along, bringing you greater discipline, a deeper practice, growth, and a fuller acceptance of yourself and others.

To give a simple example, let's say that certain food products do not agree with your body. Your intuition and your body's reaction to these foods have been telling you that these foods are not agreeable to you, yet your mind says, "Oh, just a little more." You give in to your mind but your body and intuition find a way to make you listen. The body's initial whispering will, sooner or later, turn into screams of disorder or disease. Therefore, if you choose to listen sooner rather than later, you will get the picture; you will develop a sense of discipline and be better able to avoid the potentially damaging but nonetheless lesson-filled experiences awaiting you.

As you listen more carefully and act upon your wisdom, you will realize something very important: Your body and its energy always tell you the truth. It is your rather sophisticated but undisciplined mind that takes you for a ride. Your mind will tell you that it's okay to have that bowl of ice cream, and then five minutes after you've consumed it your mind will scold you incessantly for eating it in the first place. So learn to listen to your body. It won't lie to you; it cannot do so. It's like the ignored pupil who sits at the back of the classroom, hand held steadfastly in the air, just waiting to be called on to reveal the correct answer. The mind is the child in the front shooting rubber bands at the teacher's back and then smiling innocently when the teacher turns around. Trust the voice of your body. Trust your intuition, and then use your mind's power and abilities to articulate your body's intuitive wisdom in your life.

Recommended Exercises

Connecting with the Earth
Draining Unwanted Energy from Your Body
Protecting Your Spirit
Understanding Your Body's Point of View
Clearing Energetic Impacts

6

Working with Your Body's Intelligence

I am in awe of the intelligence that drives the cells within our bodies. When I intuit cell structure I am astonished by the cells' emotional intelligence and attitude—a lot of attitude. They are sentient—a trillion little beings that tell the history of their existence. They know "things" about themselves and their neighboring cells. They can express, project, perform functions, and collect data. I have intuitively seen healthy cells next to cancer cells describing to me the differences between themselves and their unhealthy neighbors. Their animation reflects the amalgam of feelings that makes up your self-esteem. Yes, your self-esteem.

Your inner thoughts—negative, neutral, and positive—are part of the voice of your cells. They hear you and can act accordingly. If you listen to them, they can share with you what they need and what the whole of your body needs in order to achieve healing and balance—emotional, physical, energetic, and spiritual. I am convinced that you can use your cells' intelligence to help you heal.

At the age of five, I lost the belief that God was a stately grandfather sitting on a throne. Anthropomorphizing God, thinking that God had the demeanor of a human, did not make sense to me. As I grew older and pursued academics, I realized that Western views of science did not combine scientific views with religious views, especially when it came to describing human anatomy. Most academics would shrink at the thought that cells within an arm could be spoken about as having human qualities.

I still do not believe that God is like a human being. I believe God is within all beings. And I believe that a human cell's intelligence contains all that is characteristically human, energetic, and spiritual. As a medical intuitive, I have never witnessed a state of disease, in any stage of progression or regression, that did not have human characteristics and the attitude to go with it. I go into a session with a clean slate, not to objectify, compartmentalize, or create a story. What I do is read energy; and energy never lies. It is what it is, and through the use of our human language I translate the body's macro- and microcosms for the individual with whom I am working. You, too, can do the same for yourself. It takes practice, but you do have the ability to be still and neutral, and to listen.

In conjunction with the data in the energy field, the cell's behavior and attitude depict the true nature of one's physical condition. The cell membrane, in particular, is the sentient sentinel. It is a sensitive, feeling gatekeeper that has the intelligence to release, restrict, and run amok. It has enormous intelligence that can sense and manage energy, emotions, chemical toxins, and nutrients. We need to pay attention not only to our energy, our emotions, and the larger physical picture of who we are, but also to the microscopic world of our cells and their universal intelligent voice.

Your cells are the guardians and pillars of your living temple—your body. The body's intricate nature is woven together as an extraordinary matrix of form, spirit, energy, emotion, and function. Your spirit expresses through your body and personality what you are here to experience, learn, and share.

Entering the "High Heart"

A fundamental truth about being human is that, like it or not, life has a 100 percent mortality rate. It is up to you, and only you, to identify what is important and then shape your life accordingly. You are unique and possess a sacred power that is divinely entrusted to you. It is the mystical fire of your heart wherein exists the deep knowing of inner truth. Your sacred power is born from your spirit and it guides and empowers you to live the life you are destined to live. As you open your heart, you will find this seamless, divine intelligence.

This spiritual imprint is imbedded in your electromagnetic field and is reflected in the intelligence of your cells. For instance, if I were to intuitively assess the area of your body that I call the "high heart," I could hear the voice of your spirit. This area is exemplified in Christian works of art as the fiery heart of Christ or Mary. In addition, you may have seen the Buddha or other Eastern religious icons poised with a lotus flower in the center of the chest. All of these illustrate divine nature manifest within the heart. In the cells of your high heart, you can find the strongest energetic imprint of this sacred power. It holds the keys to your self-understanding and destiny. This internal chamber is a place you will enter sooner or later. It possesses the template for the spiritual calling with which you are uniquely charged in this life. As you sense your spirit through the voice and energy of this area and its cells, you will know, see, or hear whether or not you are connecting to your path.

Place your hand on your chest a few inches below your collarbone. Breathe in and out of this area. With each breath, send the intention to open up. With that, hold the intention to be at peace and awaken to who you really are. Continue to breathe in and listen.

What do you feel or sense when you do this? A lot of chatter, frustration, anger, an overwhelming life schedule? Or are peace, fulfillment, wisdom, and a sense of graceful joy present? Whatever you find, simply watch it and be aware. If there are sensations and feelings other than what you would like, change them. Breathe in the essence of peace, opening-mindedness, and soft joy. Too much joy becomes hysteria and that is not good for the heart or the soul who lives in this peaceful palace. Think of a child who is naturally sweet, curious, and filled with wonder. That softened, expansive joy will nourish your heart.

In addition, as you sense this area of the heart you can connect with the way the other organs of your body are relating to one another—energetically, physically, and spiritually. Your cells, organs, nervous system, and bodily energy are in constant communication. Their voices harmonize and tell the story of your sacred power, your life, and your wellness. It is up to you to become skilled at using your intuitive wisdom to connect. Igniting intuitive inspiration will support your mind and free will to take positive action, securing your intuitive connection with your spirit's sacred power. This will make manifest your well-being, talents, and destiny.

Spiritual, virtuous energy awakens in your life and demonstrates itself with genuine acts of kindness and generosity toward yourself and others. Courage, joy, love, compassion, and justice are some of the virtues of your sacred power. In traditional Chinese medicine these virtues are associated with the body's organs. They are in the cells of these organs and within the energy, or chi, that moves in and out of the organs.

There are negative virtues as well as positive ones. When your mind and body become saturated with negative emotions such as fear, bitterness, anger, sadness, worry, and distrust, your energy—your sacred power—is blocked. You melt into an uninspired and self-destructive life. Energetically, your body gets sluggish and you may begin to feel unwell. If your body feels unwell, your cells are feeling it too. Your mind clouds with confusion. You stop trusting yourself, and you may even begin to rely on other people's personal values and rules. Your power eventually goes out the window, along with self-esteem, spontaneity, motivation, and the ability to hear your inner wisdom.

You are entrusted with the care of your body. It is a dynamic, energetic space that will change form, ebb and flow, increase and decrease all of the time. Like any ecosystem, your energy, mind, bones, muscles, blood, and tissues are always in a state of dynamic change. Most often, these changes are subtle and seamless. They occur virtually unnoticed. On the other hand, the more awake you are to the delicate balance inherent in life, the more aware you will be of its flows. Intuitively, you can sense a change on the horizon and take preventative steps to keep your sacred power from being blocked and your body from suffering.

Because you are entrusted with your life, you are really the only one who can manage it. Your ability to support yourself is directly related to your self-esteem. That is generated and sustained by how intuitively awake, connected, and responsive you are to your spirit.

However, even if you are awake, at times not even your free will can make something different from what is occurring in the moment. You may not like what is happening in your life and you may not be able to change it at this time—or perhaps ever. It's tough to be comfortable in your own skin when you don't like what's going on with your body, your life, or your environment. But that's where you are. If you were supposed to be somewhere else, if your body was supposed to be in another condition, if you were supposed to be with someone else, you would be—that's guaranteed. You are here now. So be here. You will be able to engage your intuition more effectively and sustain inner balance even in the presence of chaos.

That is the greatest level of communication and service you can give to yourself, your body, and your life. Be here now, no matter what. It is the surest way to maintain your center and connect to your sacred power. Having your sacred power at your disposal does not ensure that life will be sweet and perfect. Life can be pretty messy. It does mean that you will be fully present to whatever is happening.

Healing Happens

So there you are, living in the moment, when a wrecking ball takes a swing at you, knocking you off your feet. Something changes in your body, and the direction of your life is suddenly altered. You become ill and get a diagnosis! Now all of your energy and the energy of those closest to you convert to single-mindedness, lasering in on your health.

Disease is complex, and can develop from myriad sources. What we do to create healing is manifold as well. To simply focus on healing your body and not your emotions or your spiritual issues is to ignore the whole of who you are. Conversely, trying to remove a disease by focusing exclusively on the energetics of what is manifest solidly in the body can be equally ineffective. I am not discounting miracles, or the anointing of the most holy in a given situation. Personally, I'm always open to the healing touch of Spirit to create both curing and healing in one sweet swoop. But the truth is that miraculous healings can be few and far between. Not everyone has that kind of lineup in their destiny. Nonetheless, let us stay open to the truth that you may be next in line for a miracle. You have to deal with where you are, what your destiny is, and what healing gift is relevant to this disorder or disease. What is miraculous to me is to be in pain or coping with a disease while still fully embracing the beauty of the world around you. That is one step shy of enlightenment.

But while you wait, it would be advantageous to be as proactive as you can for your body and that one step closer to enlightenment. I have been in the trenches of disease, both personally and professionally. As a medical intuitive and hands-on healer I have seen a woman with stage four breast cancer bring about a cure through the practice of qigong and nutrition, and then die six years later from ovarian cancer. The miracle is that she lived six years longer than traditional Western medicine had predicted. Six years! A lot of life can be lived in that amount of time.

I have seen people prevent heart attacks by listening to their inner voices—their sacred power. When the voices of their inner wisdom came into their minds, they didn't wait. They sought help from allopathic doctors and energy healers, made dietary changes, and released toxic relationships that were oppressive to their emotional and spiritual hearts. I have seen people with diabetes change not only their diets but their work schedules, types of work, and relationship boundaries. I have seen chronic rashes and nervous system issues healed through energy work on chakras to release childhood trauma. I have seen people heal their bodies while on the brink of death using Western medicine, meditation, and visualization, and then experience a deep and profound acceptance of their destiny to serve others, living a long and productive life. I have seen people heal their pain, find deep spiritual love, and physically die anyway.

Healing does not equal curing the body, at least not in all cases. Even if that is what we want, it may not be what we get. Nonetheless, you should never give up listening, being awake, and doing your best to maintain a balanced state. You can choose to spiritually and emotionally grow in whatever stage or process you may currently find yourself. The good news is that you have within you the power to sense what your body, mind, and spirit really need. This not only boosts your self-esteem and the conviction of your sense of self (which, by the way, will boost your immune system), but it allows you to follow a healthy, balanced, and free lifestyle. That is preventative medicine at its best.

You Have the Potential to Heal

The "onset" of a disease, in most cases, seems sudden. However, it is not really a sudden occurrence. The disease has been brewing chemically, energetically, and emotionally for a long time. How many people do you know, perhaps even yourself, who abuse themselves with food, lack of exercise, addictive substances, relationships, or environments because their behaviors are emotionally driven? When this occurs you are not listening to your intuition, nor are you managing you sacred power. You are not listening to your body and its cells. Your body's chemistry and cell function may have suddenly shifted and crashed; however, if you take an honest look at your experiences and emotions, you may see things that have contributed to the process.

When it comes to living with a major illness and disease, you have the potential to heal. The first rule of healing is that any harsh judgment you may be holding toward yourself or others needs to be put to rest. There will be no soft nest in which to heal if you sit on the sharp, jagged edges of judgment. As you look back to see what events might have contributed to where you are now, don't judge. If others were involved in the situation, they were most likely doing the same as you were doing: the best they could do in that moment. Simply assess and acknowledge the situation, current or past. Healing's golden rule is: Compassion and love promote healing.

Blame, criticism, and comparing your life to someone else's are derivatives of judgment. Let them go, too. Forgive. Better yet, invoke your sacred power and one of its virtues, such as courage, and walk your path with dignity and integrity. This will increase your energy and your ability to heal. Negative and fearful thoughts can cause your body's energy to become stagnant. Holding in anger or jealousy can be like holding your breath. It creates suffering and body failure. An energy leak can also develop and act like a busted water pipe hidden within a wall. You actually lose the precious vital energy force from your body; when that happens, you might as well slice off a section of your body, your self-esteem, and be less than your potential. But that is not what you are here to do.

You can stop energy leaks: First, be aware of where your energy is in the moment.

Second, ask yourself where you are receiving sensations in your body. That signal is indicative of where you need more energy and empowerment. Do you feel it in your stomach, chest, or lower back? Your stomach houses your self-esteem, self-worth, and your conviction aligned with knowing who you truly are. Your heart is the seat of your soul, an inner chamber of consciousness, and the keeper of your sacred power. Your lower back is the gateway to your life or its death; it holds your infinite power to create.

Third, sense who or what sent your energy reeling. When you are around someone and suddenly become exhausted and start yawning, I can guarantee that your energy is draining away. It is up to you to understand from which organ or energy center it is draining. When any type of energy leak occurs over time, the energy in and around your cells loses power too. Are you sick, or just sick and tired? It's your body, life, and self-worth on the line. Get in there, educate yourself in the language of energy and spirit, and engage what is challenging you. Listen to that not-so-still small voice within, and heal.

The Four Categories of Intelligences

When I intuitively assess conditions I look at four primary categories of intelligence—mechanical, emotional, energetic, and spiritual. Whether I am looking at a body from a broader perspective, as if I am standing twenty feet away, or projecting my intuition deep into a cell and its internal structures, I look at all four of these categories of intelligence.

Mechanical intelligence describes the physical body and its biochemical components. Your body's structure and movement or lack thereof are assessed from a purely mechanistic viewpoint. It is a matter-of-fact intuitive assessment of what is and isn't happening on a physical level.

Emotional intelligence is easily understood and demonstrates thoughts and behaviors (both subconscious and conscious) and how they are linked to your life experience and what is happening in the physical body. Emotional intelligence reveals itself like all levels of intelligence, meaning that it resides in both body structures and within the electromagnetic field.

Energetic intelligence addresses the various layers and levels of the electromagnetic field that surround your body, as well as the energetic permutations throughout the physical body. Each cell, organ, and body part has energy fields, grids, and connective systems. Energetic intelligence illustrates frequencies, patterns, potential areas of congestion (blockages), and density levels; all of these are important when assessing your state of well-being.

Spiritual intelligence radiates your soul's light, connecting you to your sacred power and path. It can be subtle and elusive, and often demonstrates your archetypal nature as described by psychiatrist Carl Jung. It initiates your lessons and guides your growth, and its divine spark infuses your physical body, emotions, and energetic countenance. I know you have been around people who just make you feel good, as they radiate that "something special." That is spiritual intelligence coming through. All of these categories of intelligence are interconnected. They are seamless and none of them operate independently. With the skill of intuition and a neutral but exacting mind, you can crack the code and reveal what was once mysterious and hidden.

In energy medicine, all disease states share a few commonalities. First, all diseases begin with energetic intelligence in the electromagnetic field. Whether the disease starts because of exposure to toxins in the environment, addictive habits, poor eating habits, or genetics, it first sets up its structure in this field. This is where the first signs of disease manifest. Unfortunately, not many people have the intuitive skill to sense these initial disturbances. However, with practice and dedication this ability can be developed.

Second, the four levels of intelligence I have described above are always affected by a disease. The degree to which they are affected is based on the progression of the disease. If cancer, arthritis, or another disease is developing in the field, and if you recognize it before it physically manifests, complementary medicine, psychotherapy, and nutritional cleansing can do a lot to clear it. This is early detection at its best.

Energy medicine embraces the premise that we are energy and matter; in order to live a fulfilled life and complete any necessary healing, we need to address our many facets—body, mind, and spirit. Intuitive healing is a process by which you use your intuition to access information about your body and its storehouse of data, electromagnetic energy. Using the power of your intuition, you then follow the guidance of your body and spirit and allow healing to flow through you.

In the next chapter, I would like to share with you the primary qualities that are typical of several diseases. I will focus on three of the four categories that I have just mentioned—the emotional, energetic, and spiritual levels of intelligences. At the end of each condition, I have included energetic healing slogans, which will assist those who are dealing with these issues. These slogans are also naturally preventative. Anyone can benefit from them.

A note about slogans: Often called affirmations, these slogans don't necessarily work at all times. Why is this? It is not necessarily an error on the person's part, nor is it a failure of the philosophy behind affirmations. It is simply that the body, and especially the emotional intelligence in which self-esteem lies, does not match the healing slogan. In a case such as this, little or no resonance occurs between the body's consciousness and the slogan's level of consciousness.

When I work with individuals I always ask them what their intention is. I then watch their energy field as they share that intention. My reasoning for this is that when someone says one thing but really means another, an energetic indication streams from his body, illustrating that his body and spirit don't agree with his spoken words. I see fluctuations or spikes of energy in the field indicating that there is a lack of alignment somewhere. You, too, can sense when you are saying something that is not true, that does not resonate. You can sense these spikes in your own energy field, often in the pit of your stomach or a catch in your throat.

Words hold frequencies specific unto themselves. This is true of a single word as well as a grouping of words. In regard to healing, your body must agree with the words spoken in order to move the lower frequency of the illness higher. People often say to me in their sessions, "Well, I'm saying affirmations. I have them all around my house on colorful little notes." "Great," I say. "Tell me what you're saying and I'll watch your body's energetic response in order to see if it is in alignment with your words." Most of them, I find, are not in alignment. In fact, when they speak these words their energy shrinks, or worse yet, their bodies put out an energetic and emotional rebuttal that is anything but healing. When we work with what the body really needs, rearrange the words, take away some, and add others, then there is a healing resonance.

If you want to get to the place where healing slogans such as "I love myself and I am healed" work for you, you will need to make certain that the words really resonate. You will feel a resonance or dissonance in your body. Energetic dissonance can be sensed in the body as tightness or a slight twisting feeling (as if your body cocks itself to one side and says, "That doesn't feel right"). You will mostly experience this uneasy feeling in the solar plexus, the third chakra. Obviously, if you feel dissonance, you need to rework the slogan. Instead of beginning with the slogan "I love myself" you can start with "It's okay to be me" or "It's safe to be me." Oftentimes, the word *okay* is the best place to start moving up the ramp toward the resonance of love. The word *safety* is usually in the mix as well. Sometimes it depends on how you conceptualize life. You will know what to do.

Remember, you need to feel a positive resonance in order to know that a slogan is right for you in this moment. I encourage you to play around with the healing slogans in the next chapter. See if you can intuit which work best for you. Change them around, be flexible and creative, and listen to what your inner wisdom has to say.

Recommended Exercises

Breathing In Nature's Power
Visualizing Optimal Well-being

7

Major Health Concerns: Understanding
Their Qualities and Facilitating Healing

A multitude of factors create disease. In this chapter I list several
conditions and diseases and their most prevalent energetic, emotional,
and spiritual components. There are many subtleties I cannot expand
upon within the limitations of this book. For example, genetics do cause
disease; on the other hand, most cancers and other diseases are related
to both the ingestion and poor elimination of toxins from the environment, non-nutritive foods, addictions of all kinds, and lifestyle choices.
That said, what I offer is an explanation of the common-ground qualities
within these particular conditions and diseases. The healing slogans and
other practices throughout this book have helped many people over the
years. For some, they have facilitated healing. Work with these concepts
and practices in addition to working with your physician, therapist, or
any other kind of support that feels right to you.

I have chosen these few diseases and conditions out of the myriad
problems that humanity faces because they are the most heavily

advertised in the media. Pharmaceutical companies target these conditions more than any others and I feel it is valuable to share a few insights from an energy-medicine point of view. Holistic or integrative medicine means that you use all healing methods available. These include meditation, visualization, medicines, surgery, cleansing, relocation, acupuncture, nutrition, new careers, relationship changes (mostly with one's self), and any other means that will support your health and well-being.

You will quickly find that the spiritual levels of intelligence I have noted for one disease can be applied to another. The disease to which they are attached simply signifies that this spiritual intelligence has the strongest implication for this disease. I would also suggest that you use the Clearing Energetic Impacts exercise when working with the healing slogans. If you think you are experiencing any of the issues I have listed, please be mindful and do not overthink or worry. Always seek appropriate health care in addition to doing any energetic, emotional, and spiritual work to which you are guided.

Acid Reflux

The *energetic intelligence* of acid reflux exhibits its highest concentration of energy in the solar plexus, or the third chakra, and in the electromagnetic field, where you find a chaotic flow. The energy can extend outward from the physical body two or more feet. The field bulges around the midsection, where the patterns and frequencies of this condition are held. The energy field contains particle structures that have numerous qualities, some of which are heat and cold.

Larger particles have a tendency toward damp heat while smaller particles, which suspend the larger, are dry and cold. All of the particles have a hard-rubbery quality and slightly angular shape. Their densities exemplify the extent to which this disease has affected the stomach and esophagus.

The colder particles typify the true cause of acid reflux. Point of fact: You don't get acid reflux because you have a depletion of antacids. You have a "cold" stomach because the digestive fire has gone out due to poor eating habits and a lack of digestive enzymes and stomach acid. The stomach responds by secreting more acid, and if eating habits are not changed, the condition accelerates.

The color frequencies in the energy field range from yellows and reds to darker hues of brick red and brown. Remember, more than one color frequency can always be found within the energetic construct of a condition. However, primary colors and their frequencies indicate the overall condition. Colors in the electromagnetic field and within the body will always vary due to the intensity and duration of the condition and other factors.

As you intuitively sense deeper into the body, you can approach a varying landscape. Energetic heat is present along with turbid and upward-thrusting energy. Inflammation, which is the nature of this condition, is also present and rises from the stomach into the esophageal passage. Depending on the severity of the condition, you may intuit cell damage to the lower lining of the stomach and surrounding areas. Tension and the spasmodic nature of the lower esophageal sphincter that separates the esophagus and stomach are evident.

Telescoping down into the cell structure, you will find that the cell membranes feel toxic and hot, especially in the lower section of the stomach known as the pyloric stomach. Surface cells feel both starved of and bathed in acid. Acid is supposed to be present, of course, but in a balanced way. Typically, it is underproduced. The stomach quickly makes more as a result of this underproduction, and then an overproduction suddenly floods the stomach. Energetically, the cells are bright red with a thin, marbled coating of black and yellow around them. The cardiac, or upper, stomach's cells are less red and the surrounding colors are typically grayish-red and mauve. These cell membranes appear slightly heartier and less damaged than those of the pyloric stomach cells.

The *emotional intelligence* demonstrates an emotionally reactive nature, even if the emotions are not expressed outwardly. More often than not, this condition results from a lack of connection between the emotional self and the physical body. Often, a strong emotional energy in the third chakra that says "I am invincible" can result in behavior that says "I can eat anything; I can put up with anything or anyone." A thought form such as "I will not be denied" has the same effect.

Cells typically show the emotions of worry, being overwhelmed, frustration, or repressed anger. You will often find anger that specifically stems from feelings of injustice and disappointment within the cell membrane of the stomach. "I can't take this anymore" is a common cry that began long before the condition surfaced.

The *spiritual intelligence* is about learning to keep things in balance and perspective, continuing to self-inspire and -motivate. The shadow teachers of this condition are feelings of being overwhelmed and acting out with overeating, overwork, or any other "overage." If you have this condition, learning to honor and respect yourself is the spiritual gift. As you honor and respect yourself, you will gain spiritual clarity and understand your destiny. No longer will you push yourself, your body, or anyone else.

This respect is born from an understanding that life does change, and that all you can do is listen deeply to your rhythms and follow the beat of your own drum. You will no longer try to conform to others' schedules or make them conform to yours. Simply listen and do your best.

Patience is essential as you learn to let go of things or people whom you cannot control. Not stuffing down your emotions is also an important spiritual and energetic metaphor for this condition. As you begin to listen to the physical, reactive anger of your stomach and become more careful about what you put into your body, you will also begin to care more about the physical and emotional environments in which you place yourself. Self-satisfaction will begin to arise from taking these small, inwardly directed steps. What is eliminated is the previously pressure-filled mind ruled by the tendencies of perfectionism, anger, and fear.

The spiritual intelligence of this condition teaches you that you may not be in control, but you always have a choice about how you respond and care for yourself. You become accountable for yourself because you are the only one who can really choose for yourself. You learn to honor your dreams and goals. And by listening deep within to your wisdom, you know your true destiny. Consequently, you begin to walk along with life, not chase it down like a wild steer. Nor do you run away from all that is yours.

Balancing Slogans

I love and respect my body.

I move easily with the changes in life. (Work up to the phrase "I love change.")

I honor my personal vision.

I am kind to myself.

I am calm.

I feel supported.

Breathing deeply into my body, I calmly remember my destiny and know that all is well. (Say this one even if your personal mission is not yet clear. It will become so.)

Anxiety

The *energetic intelligence* of anxiety is primarily centered in the first and third chakras. Its emotional emphases are fear of life's unpredictability and the feeling of a lack of safety (first chakra), along with an insufficiency of self-confidence and personal esteem manifested as fear (third chakra). Depending on the intensity of the anxiety, varying degrees of instability and a lack of energy will appear in both of these chakras.

The energetic structure of the first and third chakras wavers as tension and anxiety rise and fall within the person. (Breathing exercises will help calm this.) There are also spikes of energy that create concentric rings and erratic patterns in the energy field and the chakras. At the peak of an anxiety attack, for instance, the once-smooth and consistent oscillations of the chakra and field are interrupted. The first chakra's energy drops away from the body, literally whooshing downward. It is the energetic equivalent of "having the rug pulled out from under you."

The structure of the first chakra is radically altered in an anxiety attack, so much so that all senses tell the body and mind that something is going to falter. Worst-case scenarios include having a heart attack, passing out, or failing physically in some other way. These sensations are felt running throughout the body; failure is on the horizon. This experience is accentuated if a person has faced some type of overwhelming or life-threatening stressor, such as post-traumatic stress syndrome. The energetic memory of these stresses activates and adds its force to the current attack.

The third chakra loses power in a downward and outward motion. It descends through the energy system and joins in the downward thrust of the first chakra. It can also shoot out the front of the body, leaving one with a fluttering, queasy stomach or nausea. The back of the third chakra is often shut down, as there is little or no willfulness left from which to draw. The third chakra matches the energy of the first chakra's destabilized pattern.

The third chakra does not suffer the same sudden loss of energy as does the first chakra, but it is depleted nonetheless. It becomes confused as it tightens and expands in unpredictable patterns, undulating to find some safe place of equanimity or balance. It tightens to conserve energy, unlike the first chakra, which opens wide and elongates, creating the feeling of losing control.

The energetic recovery time from a panic attack ranges from thirty minutes to an hour or more; during this time the body begins to draw energy from other internal and external sources and systems in order to rebalance and stabilize. These internal systems are other chakra centers, energy pathways such as nadis, organs, muscle tissues, and bones. External sources include other people's energy, food and water, sunlight, any form of precipitation, trees, bodies of water, or any aspect of nature. Mountains naturally have tremendous energy and strength, but not everyone lives near a mountain. The earth's grounding energy is the key to refueling and reestablishing the first and third chakras.

In the body's electromagnetic field, the energy of anxiety is characterized by fluctuating, short spikes of energy. These spikes occur under several circumstances. For example, when someone is nervous or anxious, the field will spike and send off energetic flares, which can be either hot or cold. The length of these spikes will vary based on the intensity of the panic attack and the level of stress hormones released in the body. Typically, they are two to ten inches in length but can reach up to eighteen inches and indicate moderate to extreme emotion. The spikes' temperatures demonstrate extremes as well. In other words, they can be very hot or merely warm, cold, or cool.

An irony of this condition is that the structure of the field is both nimble and rigid. Again, extremes present themselves. The nimble nature is due to the fact that most people dealing with anxiety are sensitive and are energetically and emotionally quick to react. They are empathic and feel other people's energy and feelings very easily. There is not an empathic person alive who has not cried during a Hallmark commercial or the evening news. And their blessing can be a curse as well until they learn how to energetically anchor themselves, place trust in their heightened sensitivities, know that they are safe, and reroute their empathic nature into a solid gift that supports their existence and their path of service.

In addition, when someone is dealing with either a general sense or sudden onset of anxiety, you can intuitively see or sense the person's spirit in a state of anticipation, ready to jump out of the physical body if anything or anyone perceived as threatening comes near. Because breathing is often shallow and ineffective, the etheric layer of the energy field is compressed around the upper torso of the body, while it can become virtually nonexistent from the waist down. (The etheric energy body typically extends from just within the physical surface of the body outward approximately twelve to fourteen inches. It is the densest part of the electromagnetic field and is also the template for the physical body.)

This demonstrates a lack of grounding, and as is the case with their physical counterparts, there is an energetic strain on the adrenal glands. The adrenals are known as the "the root of life" in traditional Chinese medicine. When they are in balance, the virtue that resonates throughout them is joy. Conversely, when they are out of balance, as occurs during anxiety, the virtues are those of fear and ungrounded energy. It may be difficult to view fear as a virtue, but fear often has merit in one's life as a teacher and bringer of lessons. Think of it this way: There is no good or bad in joy or fear; there is only direction toward or away from one or the other. Both have potential lessons, and therefore both hold merit. Merit is virtuous. When you think of emotions in this way, you are less affected by them and remain in a balanced state of simple happiness. After all, hysterical joy can quickly lead to tears, anger, sadness, and fear. Emotions create a dynamic flow and disarm their seemingly negative effects by flowing with them.

The *emotional intelligence* indicates that the person is empathic and sensitive. The organs in the solar plexus (third chakra) hold emotions that reflect an inner questioning about the person's true nature: "Who am I?" "What am I here for?" and "When is this going to get better?" We all ask those questions at some point in our lives, but anxiety constantly runs them through the emotional intelligence of the cells.

Since people suffering from anxiety can easily pick up others' feelings, their emotional intelligence gets confused and sometimes has difficulty separating others' ideas from their own. A cry deep inside the body arises from setting aside what is wanted in life. A course is set for a never-ending search for acceptance, which can only be found within. Feelings of uncertainty, confusion, fear, and hopelessness arise because grounding, a solid sense of knowing who the self is, self-acceptance, and self-love are absent.

Because a person is often afraid that people will see who she really is, even the wonderful things about her, the emotional intelligence of anxiety may not let her see her own gifts. There is an outer life of posturing and an inner life that resembles both a scared cat up in a tree and someone trying to talk it down—all at the same time.

The *spiritual intelligence* and the message around anxiety is that through life's experiences a person will gain a stronger, more wakeful presence of self, owning who she is, gifts and all. She develops courage as she steps through each anxiety attack. The energy of self-esteem slowly builds, cultivating personal conviction from which happiness will eventually arise. As she gains this certainty, she becomes comfortable within her skin. The eventual ownership of spiritual gifts and human talents creates the mosaic of her life's purpose.

Balancing Slogans

I am courageous.

I am confident.

I know who I am.

I am okay. (I am safe.)

I trust my body.

I am healthy.

I live happily.

*With every breath I feel my spirit is
fully grounded in my body,
igniting my gifts and purpose.*

Arthritis

The *energetic intelligence* connected with arthritis has alternating areas of hot and cold, similar to a patchwork quilt. Undulating bands of energy fluctuate in the field. They are present within the areas that hold and radiate warmth, much like heat rising from a desert road in the summer. Spikes in the electromagnetic field are present and vary in height according to the degree of pain. Pockets of stagnated energy form around affected joints. You can sense the heat and moisture that are also in the cell structure.

The energetic colors are variations of red, brown, and yellow. Darker hues of these colors can indicate a greater degree of severity and the impact of arthritis within the joints. (This is true for most conditions. Darker colors typically indicate a denser concentration of particles in a diseased state. The denser the particles, dark or light, the more the condition or consciousness has settled into the body.)

These colors, fluctuations, and spikes of energy exist within the specific layer of the energy field that surrounds the body known as the etheric field.

With arthritis, secondary areas of energetic stagnation can be detected all around the body. These areas are indicative of compromised muscular structure due to the limited movement associated with arthritic conditions. For instance, if there is arthritis demonstrating in the knees, it can have neuromuscular effects throughout the legs and even the muscles of the hips. This energy characteristically positions itself on the surface of the body and extends outward to about six inches. It can extend out more dramatically; however, pain medications tend to reduce the extension of such energy by reducing the pain.

Deeper into the bones and joints, you still find hot and cold energy pockets. Joint fluids tend to be hot and you can sense the chemical imbalance that is indicative of degeneration or, at a minimum, the directional movement toward it. All of these indicators vary depending on the severity of the case.

The structural density of bone and cartilage can decrease, and you can intuitively see a more lace-like structure as this occurs. The greater the density loss, the more holes in the lace, so to speak.

The *emotional intelligence* is exacerbated by tension in the ligaments and the attachment points of muscles where they connect to the joints. As is the case with many chronic conditions, it turns into a "Catch-22." The emotion that is usually found within arthritis is a deep internal tension constructed from fear, inflexibility, and uncertainty. Fear of moving forward, the inability to release old hurts that have turned inward, and confusion about the direction of a person's life can be found in the heat and chemical imbalances of the joints and surrounding tissues. Even if they are genetically driven, these emotions can take up housekeeping in the body.

The *spiritual intelligence* is found within the very core of the bones and has a literal meaning and purpose in the body's joints. Freedom of movement, freedom to be oneself spiritually, and freedom to creatively express one's self are the core teachings. Having fluid joy and creativity in one's life is the most significant spiritual lesson of arthritis. Letting go of past emotional pain is not easy to do if one is in chronic pain with tender muscles or gnarled joints. However, the spiritual growth that comes from this type of work is immeasurable.

In learning these lessons for yourself, you look at the attachments to beliefs and issues that currently hold or have held you back from your dreams and goals. You need to ask what ideas, values, things, and situations are worth holding onto. Only you can decide as you reach deep inside to your bones and find what moves you and how you are to express your dynamic spirit.

Balancing Slogans

I live in a state of joy.

I am open to life.

I freely express my creative spirit.

I feel joy in my bones.

No matter what, I love my life.

As I breathe in, energy spirals around my joints and bones,
allowing me to be healed, open, and free.

Cancer

A common link to all disease states is that of its energetic beginning. The *energetic intelligence* of cancer begins in the electromagnetic field.

Cancer's unique quality of energy manifests as infinitesimal particles within the field. Although most diseases begin as particles, cancer particles are distinguished by irregular angles that are oddly geometric. They are also dark in color, glossy, and concretized.

As this energy builds in the electromagnetic field, the energy centers (chakras and meridians) begin to become obstructed and the flow of energy to the organs becomes restricted. This process is the energetic path of any disease; however, cancer in particular creates some of the most restrictive blocks. Just as a cancer cell pushes healthy cells out of the way in search of more blood to sustain its embryonic growth, so too does its energetic characteristic. These dark, shiny particles overtake the healthy, vibrant structures of the electromagnetic field, obstructing the flow of energy and creating congestion.

Cancer's particles, whether you look at them in the electromagnetic field or in the physical body, are typically variants of black, red, and gray. They range in hue and intensity depending on the cancer's severity and progression. The texture of cancerous energy is sticky, and becomes progressively concretized as it takes hold in the body.

The initial particles hold an *emotional intelligence* that is fiercely independent and rebellious. As the potential for the manifestation of the disease progresses, the particles increase in density and begin to coagulate, thus lowering the frequency of the field. Consequently, various bodily systems, including the immune system, weaken, and one's overall sense of physical well-being diminishes.

It is within this independence and rebellion that you can intuitively find the core issues of cancer—fear, deep sadness, and grief. Anger is certainly present within cancer; however, there is an overlay of sadness and grief. The immune system is associated with the first and third chakras and has strong connections to the adrenals and to the endocrine system in general. The endocrine system is closely associated with the nonphysical chakra system. This is why, energetically speaking, cancer shows up in various chakra regions that correspond to endocrine glands and other body organs shown in table 1:

Table 1

Endocrine Gland	Chakra
Hypothalamus/pituitary	Seventh and sixth chakras
Thyroid	Fifth chakra
Adrenals	Third chakra
Ovaries/testes	Second and first chakras
Body Organ	
Brain	Seventh and sixth chakras
Mouth/throat/lung	Fifth chakra
Lung	Fifth and fourth chakras
Liver/stomach/pancreas/ gall bladder/spleen/kidney	Third chakra
Uterus/ovary/bladder/prostate	Second (with connections to first chakra)
Small and large intestines	First, second, and third chakras

The *spiritual intelligence* of cancer is a perception of being afraid and restricted in life. Seated in both the unconscious and conscious minds, feelings of being fearful, cut off from love, or unable to truly express one's uniqueness are found within the cells, the energy field, and energy system lines (meridians and chakras). Some part of the self has been denied. Oftentimes, the spiritual gift of cancer shows us where we have been hiding our true feelings.

The rebel in us all is a powerful ally. It is the primary fuel for our creativity. As the rebel matures and marshals self-esteem, it turns into the producer and generates our success and achievement. The more mature and balanced the rebel becomes, the more clarity, confidence, and success enter our lives.

Balancing Slogans

I have found my voice and easily express my true nature.

I am okay.

I am safe.

I am loved and feel love deep within.

With every breath I take I feel the joy, love, and light of God flowing into every cell in my body.

Depression

In general, *energetic intelligence* identifies when our chemistry is out of balance. We know that in order to maintain wellness, it is critical to maintain this balance. The energy of depression really does appear as the "dark cloud" to which people often refer, and this particular con-figuration of the dark cloud does indicate chemical imbalances. A gray cloud of particles surrounds the body. One of the interesting qualities of these particles is that when you go into them intuitively, they will disappear. All I can see is a dark ring around the particle structure. The rest of it turns into a clear mass, or the particle disappears completely, as if for some reason it doesn't want to be seen. These particles are soft, malleable, and quick to move when I sweep an energetic healing hand through the field.

Particles can be highly concentrated over the heart or solar plexus area (fourth and third chakras). Even if someone is simply holding onto depressed emotions for a short period of time, you can see the darkness arising from or hovering over these chakras, in particular the heart chakra. Chronic chemical depression holds stagnation in the third chakra and within the sixth and seventh. Short-term depression is more heart chakra oriented, and typically clears after some kind of expression of anger or grief.

With chronic chemical depression, the outward energy is as described above. Going deeper into the physical structure, you find myriad issues. Typically, the adrenals have a sluggish grid of energy around them with disappointment and forlorn emotional aspects. The same is true for the thyroid and the cells and lining of the stomach. The gut-associative lymphatic tissue is typically grayish-red and at times can indicate some inflammation in the ducts.

Going more intensely into cell structure, we find receptor sites on the cell membranes that have a depressed, childlike rebellious nature. Most are closed. They are just too sad and stubborn to open. The same is true for the neurological receptor sites in the brain. After a while they lose their rebellious nature and just go to sleep. Even the mitochondria within the cells seem to lose their energetic spark, and their emotional intelligence has the presence of "just not knowing what to do." With the energy of depression, emotional energy feels lost.

The old saying "depression is anger turned inward" reflects the *emotional intelligence*. Without disputing this statement, I want to add, however, that this inward anger is a result of not knowing who one is and the inability to exercise one's sense of self.

Feelings of being controlled by others or by circumstances are present, especially in the heart and liver. If you are depressed, these emotions exist because you don't feel you have the ability to control yourself. They manifest energetically as congestion in the solar plexus and chest (third and fourth chakras respectively). In addition, both centers can have countless energetic cords extending in all directions. These cords are connections to others, past or present. Energetically, you're still tied to another's energy or specific life events. This creates a constant energetic and emotional loop—the incessant negative tape that runs through the mind. Remember, a thought of your past is just a thought and not the event itself. Release it emotionally and find balance.

The solar plexus and the heart chakra are the primary holders of emotional pain. Worry, anger, and the depletion of joy in one's life are evident. There is a repressive energy that says you may never be able to achieve what you desire. The past keeps emotionally looping around in the body, energy, and mind. When these emotions go back and forth for an extended period of time and the energy is never released, grief starts to enter into the mix, solidifying the dark cloud around you. It is that emotional energetic component of grief that seals the depression and concretizes as such in the body and mind.

The emotional intelligence is primarily embedded within the organs of the third chakra: small intestinal tract, liver, heart, and spleen. The gut's lymphatic system, where 90 percent of serotonin is made, is affected as well. The body cries for something, anything, or anyone able to offer a sense of purpose, love, and satisfaction. Deep emotional wounds, sometimes over little things, have festered for a long time.

I agree with the hereditary aspects of depression and anxiety. In addition, energetic and emotional heredity is just as valid from an energy-medicine point of view. People prone to depression and anxiety are typically empathic and feel things easily and deeply. That, too, is passed down from generation to generation. To harness the power of this gift is the task, as it is the spiritual blessing of an empath.

"Life gets to be about you," says the *spiritual intelligence* of depression. Not that you are a narcissist, but because you are the only one in your own skin. You can give yourself permission to feel your feelings and follow your dreams as long as you maintain a sense of accountability for your actions.

Self-love is the antidote and the gatekeeper to freeing yourself from depression. It is true that most spiritual lessons are delivered paradoxically. For instance, you know that you need to love yourself and know who you are, but you *don't!* Getting clear on your values and what is important to you and never compromising those deeper truths can bring you home. Holding a deep conviction of the preciousness of your life opens the gate and allows you to enter into the spiritual garden of the Self.

Balancing Slogans

I know what is important to me.

It's okay to be me.

Loving is easy.

I am comfortable with my power.

I feel joy deep inside.

With each breath I feel my true nature emerging.

Type 2 Diabetes

Energetic grids exist around all organs, bones, and tissue. These grids remain when there is a developing condition or even a full-blown disease. Like the overall intuitive within, these energetic grids tell a story; they hold data. The energy patterns around the pancreas share the story of diabetes and its progression. With type 2 diabetes the *energetic intelligence* rests mostly within the electromagnetic field, the second, third, fourth, and fifth chakras, as well as around the pancreas, spleen, stomach, and upper digestive tract.

These specific energetic patterns begin as a buildup of energetic congestion that forms slightly left of center around the midsection of the body. One of the interesting dynamics of diabetes is that the particles of the disease simultaneously exhibit the energies of both expansion and contraction.

The expanded energy around the solar plexus is due to the growing congestion and the forthcoming potential of the disease. As you intuitively peer into this configuration of energy, you can sense concave and contracted energy that has an inward-drawing motion. This is due to the stress on the pancreas, inflammation, and the lack of digestive enzymes. It indicates diminished life-force energy that is being drained by attacks from the immune system on the tiny cells of the Islets of Langerhans, which hinders the pancreas's ability to adequately produce the hormone insulin. As the disease approaches and progresses, all of the organs associated with digestion and assimilation suffer both energetically and chemically.

The energetic colors and vibrancy of the pancreas begin to dim and darken. Gray to dark charcoal-colored particles begin to form in the field around the midsection of the body. Heat, typically red, yellow, and gray, begins to radiate and be held within the pancreas. With the progression of the condition, it moves into the duodenum, the first section of the small intestinal tract.

The stronghold for patterns of *emotional intelligence* is located in the spleen, stomach, upper digestive tract, and pancreas. The emotional intelligences of diabetes are worry, projecting worst-case scenarios, overthinking, and overplanning. People are unique, and to describe the emotional/energetic patterns of type 2 diabetes—or any disease—in a linear way is risky, since none of this happens energetically in a linear fashion. However, it is the only way to articulate the stages and patterns that occur in accordance with energy medicine.

Over a lifetime, sensitive people, who may hold in their emotions, receive deep energetic hits of information about the others for whom they care. These hits can be related to family, work, or any issue in life about which they feel deeply and which they hold in at the same time as they try to figure it out. The primary energetic target of this incoming information is the solar plexus. The bodily message they feel is that "something is out of balance and needs to be done for this person or project. I can't stand conflict. I'll fix it!"

After initially impacting the third chakra, the energetic signals move to the second chakra, the center of creativity and problem solving. Lo and behold, potential resolutions come forward through this part of the energy system and then move into the conscious energy of the heart chakra. "Does this feel good? Does this not?" are the queries of the heart.

If it "feels good" the fifth chakra comes on board and expresses the resolution or activity. If it doesn't "feel good" in the heart, the energy travels back down to the second chakra, and another solution is ground out. While that grinding is going on in the second chakra, the third chakra and heart chakra are starting to build the energy and emotions of worry, grief, or panic. This worsens until the second chakra comes up with the solution. Often, the resolution comes at the expense of one person trying to solve the problem for another, trying to make the other person's life safer, sweeter, and less stressful. That is the key emotional intelligence that resides in type 2 diabetes: making life better for others at the expense of one's own life-force energy. Secondary intelligence is holding emotions in and not verbally processing issues in a reasonable manner. Generous, sensitive people holding in their hurt, anger, and disappointment about not having their life to live are common sufferers of this condition.

If you have type 2 diabetes, you will find that the *spiritual intelligence* and lessons embedded in it are about self-trust and supporting your emotional needs with healthy boundaries that honor yourself. Calming thoughts projected into the pancreas, spleen, and stomach are beneficial. Invoking peace and the courage to let others go is essential. Listening to your body's needs will create a deeper sense of trust. Personal freedom and a sense of sweetness derived from inner happiness are the spiritual sinews of this condition. When you have better boundaries, you make better choices for yourself in all areas of life—career, intimate relationships, money, and nutrition. You trust yourself to manage your emotional/energetic boundaries by knowing what is yours to deal with and what belongs to others. This hones the power of the third chakra. You give your second-chakra energy a break and don't try to fix the world, especially at the expense of your life or livelihood.

Balancing Slogans

I am peaceful.

I trust God to guide my life.

I know what is mine to deal with.

It's my journey to live to my fullest capacity.

I freely express my playful spirit.

I have healthy boundaries.

I breathe in healing golden light,
filling my body with deep knowing and trust.

Fibromyalgia and Chronic Fatigue Syndrome

These immune-system disorders are closely linked energetically. They are different diseases; however, many people suffer from both conditions simultaneously. From an energetic perspective, both of these conditions demonstrate what I call "dirty energy." If you have ever seen the *Peanuts* character Pig Pen, the little boy who carries a cloud of dust around his body, this is what I'm talking about. While this descriptor of *energetic intelligence* is no personal, hygienic, or psychological refection on anyone who has this condition, it is the simplest way to describe its energetic structure. The dirt-like particles of these diseases surround the person's body in a free-floating manner, condensing and dispersing with the progression or regression of these conditions.

The energetic structures of these particles are round with undulating surfaces. Some are clear with dark outer edges and soft, rubbery texture. Other particles are black and harder with rough and spiky surfaces. The more intense the disease, the more resistant this rubbery quality becomes. This texture is found within the particles of the field, as well as around the energy grids of the body's cells. Because digestive issues often accompany these conditions, the cells in the intestinal tract also reflect this energetic quality. Hormones are also strongly affected by this condition.

With these diseases there is little energetic ebb and flow within the field or the body's internal energetic systems. This reflects in four of its primary systems: the nervous system, endocrine system (which regulates and secretes hormones), neuromuscular system, and digestive system. A person with these conditions may often be energetically sensitive, and extremely chemically sensitive to foods, scents, household chemicals in clothing and building materials, and petrochemicals.

The two diseases differ energetically in the energy field. Fibromyalgia has more heat associated with it, and this heat is also found in the energy field, the muscles, and within the cytoplasm (the fluid inside the cell walls). Chronic fatigue syndrome, on the other hand, creates weakness in the section of the electromagnetic field that processes our emotions; appropriately, this section of the energy field is called the emotional field. These pockets of weakened energy have less density than other sections. Therefore, they energetically demonstrate a lack of physical and emotional stamina. These holes are literal depletion points and mirror the emotional depletion that builds prior to and during the course of the disease.

Energetically, both fibromyalgia and chronic fatigue syndrome solidify a tight barrier around the physical body. This barrier ranges from four to ten inches as it extends away from the body, and is the restrictive force on healthy energy. This, again, reflects the lack of ebb and flow. I have found that the practices of tai chi and qigong, along with nutrition and traditional Chinese medicine techniques such as acupuncture, assist people with these conditions in making headway once they begin to regain health. The Running the Rainbow exercise located in the Appendix has been reported by clients to be very helpful for these conditions.

The *emotional intelligences* of these conditions range from a fearful grip and shutting one's energy completely down to a gradual release of this oppressive hold and then opening with optimism. The emotions often found around the cells and glands of the body are of a heightened state of awareness and reactivity. Endocrine gland cells are emotionally hyper-vigilant, marked by the paradoxical postures of lack of boundaries and timidity. It is as if the energetic boundaries of the sensitive person have failed. She wants to engage in life and feel well, but her body just says, "No way! I'm not going out there! And don't let anyone in!" The organs of the third chakra—liver, gallbladder, kidney, spleen, stomach, pancreas, and the small intestinal tract—can all hold similar emotional intelligences. Often it is a voice of sensitivity to stimuli, making the cells and tissue push with the posture of the overachiever and perfectionist.

Cellular emotions display an exhausted intelligence, but like honorable little solders, they keep pushing on. Cells give off energetic bursts, as if they are giving the body's systems their very last drop of energy. The mitochondria within the cell, which perform a multitude of cell functions, are marked by a confused state of not knowing what to do. They still work, but not optimally.

The nervous system is postured as if under attack. Stress-burdened, the emotional and chemical feedback loop from the nervous system to the endocrine system feels as if it never gets a break. Toxins literally build up in the body from stress hormones and have nowhere to go. The energy field and tissues of the body scream with exhaustion as if to say, "I can't give one more ounce of me, because there's nothing left to give!"

Lessons imbued in the *spiritual intelligence* are about personal power that involves balance, boundaries, and knowing the line of demarcation between perfectionism and impeccability.

If you experience fibromyalgia or chronic fatigue syndrome, it is essential to create healthy boundaries with whatever and whoever is toxic and draining in your life. It may mean that you need to physically move away from a chemically toxic environment. A career change might be in order, as the current one is making you ill from the inside out. Your personality may push and push and push and you don't listen to your own body's cries as stress chemicals build, eventually breaking down the endocrine system. If you are a very sensitive person, your body could be saturated with the energetic, emotional pain and suffering of those people whom you have helped.

Boundaries are a result of knowing who you are on a values level. What do you value? Your body, life, health, creativity, honesty, love, and fun are all values. Only you and your spiritual intelligence know what yours are.

Knowing your values naturally provides a set of personal rules. If you discard or step on your values, or let someone else do so, you are blowing off your personal rules. That's a deal breaker, and at times, a body breaker. Discovering your values will lead you to your personal rules. They generate boundaries. So what are your values? What rules come from them and what boundaries are there to support their integrity? It's a circle. Break a link in it and there will be little or no harmony. Spiritually speaking, balance and harmony are the gifts of these conditions.

Balancing Slogans

I make good choices for myself, my body, and my spirit.

I honor my values.

I know what is important to me.

I trust myself.

I am loyal to myself and my needs.

I am compassionate with myself and others.

I am passionate about my life.

As I breathe into my body I am refueled by the harmonious connection I have to God and nature. I know and trust myself.

High Blood Pressure

The fourth chakra, the third chakra, and the etheric field—the energy field that is closest to the physical body—all hold the *energetic intelligence* for high blood pressure. The energy appears full and dense in the top half of the body when high blood pressure is present. The field also tends to narrow from the waist down, giving the etheric field a "light bulb" shape. Medication reduces the upper extension of the field. Nonetheless, as you intuitively enter into the body and sense the interior of the heart chamber you can feel the tension. In and around the arterial structures, those extending from the top of the heart especially exhibit this tension.

Going more deeply into the arterial walls, you can intuit the depletion of elasticity within them. Whatever is occurring within the outer layer, in this case the arterial wall, you can at times sense in the smaller structures. For example, there are tension, a sense of pressure, and rigidity in the field as well as within the cell membranes of the heart and arterial walls.

The colors in the field and around the heart are typically in a band from red to orange to yellow. The more uncontrolled the pressure is, the darker the hue of each color. It is helpful to intuitively scan the kidneys when high blood pressure is present to see if any corresponding levels of pressure or loss of elasticity are reflected there as well.

It is equally important not to intuitively confuse the strength of the heart muscle with increased pressure. You must "talk" to the heart's muscles and its cells to fully understand if the sensation of strength is coming from a physical/pressure issue or an emotional component. Both can be present in high blood pressure. You never want to make any assumptions without "looking" at all the pieces. Remember, when using intuition you do not generate or embellish upon what is happening. You simply read energy and interpret your findings as best you can.

We know that stress and being overweight are both causes of high blood pressure. The *emotional intelligence* of this condition calls on us to examine our emotional buildup. Overthinking, overwhelm, and worry and resulting stress cause the body's energy to rise. If there is no relaxation or letting go of that stress, the energy cannot release the upward-thrusting, trapped energy. It cannot move downward.

The emotional intelligence of high blood pressure is usually seated in the back of the heart chakra and indicates that we have lost touch with our deeper emotions.

Whether it is caused by holding emotions or holding weight, high blood pressure is about holding. Our *spiritual intelligence* beckons us to let go of control and find inner peace and balance. These are the spiritual lessons of high blood pressure. Movement in any area of life in which we feel restricted is the spiritual antidote.

Balancing Slogans

I feel freedom deep inside.

I take life one thing at a time.

I hold gentleness in my heart.

Gratitude and appreciation fill my heart.

When I breathe deeply into my chest, I feel joy and reverence for my life and for the world around me.

High Cholesterol

The seat of *energetic intelligence* for this condition is in the liver, small intestine, and heart—the third and fourth chakras respectively. Particles of congested energy first begin to build around the midsection of the body, slightly right of center. This is the first indication that there is a potential stagnation problem both in the energy of the liver and within the liver itself. The liver's texture remains the same, relatively healthy; however, you can intuitively sense the congestion in the internal tissue, especially the far right side of the liver. The energetic grid around the liver feels thick and sluggish, and over time that energy spreads to the small intestinal tract as well as the stomach.

In the stomach, heat begins to form and pass back toward the liver. The small intestine cannot escape the increase in heat, and so the cells along the inner wall of the jejunum, the second section of the small intestinal tract, build up a thick energy grid as well. Nutritional absorption becomes compromised.

The heart's "attitude" should be checked; if it does not reflect the tension and congestion in the liver, you can usually predict that the arteries will clear as well. Nonetheless, the arterial passages must be intuitively scanned, as their internal cell walls can hold the same tension and congestion energetically as the liver and small intestine. If the arterial passages are clear, you can focus healing measures on the liver and small intestinal tract with diet and exercise. Herbs, energy work, and supplements are available to help lower cholesterol. Statins are commonly used in Western medicine and are effective, although they tend to build up more heat in the liver, thus creating problems and adding to the congestive cycle.

When we bury our true nature or push ourselves too much, our liver pays the price. Often associated with the *emotional intelligence* of anger, the liver's deep emotional energy is that of knowing and doing who we really are. When we restrict ourselves from living our inner joy, or circumstances make us feel that way, we build up emotional congestion in the liver.

Being able to take the time for spiritual work within is the basis of the *spiritual intelligence*. Life gets so busy. It can also be sloppy, challenging us in ways we hadn't expected. We push, thinking we have to be on the edge and go, go, go all the time. Yes, life forces us to do that, but these demands are based solely on the attachments to what we think we should have and who we think we are. A wise person takes the time—a month, week, or day—to reflect. Such times of reflection clear congestion energetically, emotionally, physically, and certainly spiritually.

In traditional Chinese medicine the liver is known as the general, the taskmaster who leads all the other organs. Its energy guides and supports the flow of energy throughout the body, assimilating, cleansing, and purifying. That is the spiritual lesson behind this condition. If your cholesterol is high, you have work to do, but you must rest as well. Internal searching that leads to the discovery of your true nature is the shining gift presented in this condition. Lower your cholesterol and you lower the resistant and attendant congestion to being who you are. The liver's energetic spiritual gift allows you to find your gifts and use them accordingly. That is the mission with which you have been charged. As the liver gives "orders" to the other organs, so must you take to heart the spiritual orders for your life.

Balancing Slogans

I own my power.

I love my life.

I feel peace and happiness deep inside.

I know what I am here to do.

I love to share my gifts with others.

I do my best with what God has given me.

As I breathe deeply into my precious body, I feel relaxation, calm, and satisfaction. I am in harmony with my world.

Irritable Bowel Syndrome

Irritable Bowel Syndrome (IBS) creates unsuspecting and quick fluctuations in the electromagnetic field. This reactivity in the first and third chakras is the primary *energetic intelligence* and driver of this condition.

For the most part, the energy field looks normal. There is good density, a wide girth, full coverage from above the head to below the feet. There can be a slight narrowing from the waist down, but this depends on the severity of the condition. The energy field closest to the body—the etheric field—signals that there is an issue. In addition, the third and first chakras are weak and reactive and carry a sense of vulnerability. Short, jagged spikes can also characterize this condition, although they are not always present.

The colon and parasympathetic nervous system are the primary physiological points of concern, along with the lungs, stomach, spleen, and kidneys. Energetically, there is pressure in the form of anticipatory stress on the adrenals and nervousness in the third chakra. These organs show energetic weakness and vulnerability, and have less energetic density. Their energetic grids are hyperreactive to stimuli of all kinds.

The *emotional intelligence* points to a sense of unwanted vulnerability within the energy fields and organ tissues. A perceived loss of personal authority and control is present as well, especially in the stomach, small intestine, and colon. Fairness and justice, or the lack thereof, are often woven within the field. I would not say it is a victim mentality; there is a sense of idealism and innocence associated with it. It is more like a feeling that all things should be fair, and they are not; therefore, one doesn't feel safe. Instead, one feels is as if anything could happen at any moment.

There are both emotional strengths and qualities of vulnerability. It is one of the more paradoxical emotional intelligences that I have seen. The body can handle it, and then it suddenly can't. Grief plays a part within the body's cells as well as the energy field, but is not the first emotional intelligence to arrive on the scene. It is secondary to the perceived loss of authority and control over what one wants in life.

The spiritual power of impermanence is the *spiritual intelligence* connected with this disorder. Impermanence can mean what the dictionary implies: that all things change. However, there is a deeper spiritual meaning behind this term that comes from Buddhism; impermanence has more to do with the force that animates all things in an ever-changing manner than with the surface, recognizable acts of change.

We are growing older and so our faces change. That is surface impermanence. The deeper meaning is one of a pervasive animator that is the essence of change. Things change because change is the very nature, essence, and purification of life.

To trust in this ever-changing flow is to be fully present in the moment and let all things be just as they are. When we "let go" of things, this is not the same as releasing all of our relationships and possessions, simply possessiveness. It is attachment that brings suffering and the animating force of impermanence that moves things all of the time. With IBS, the spiritual intelligence conveys trust in the ever-changing nature of reality and life.

Balancing Slogans

I am safe in this world.

I am comfortable with change.

I am peaceful.

I respond with ease to my changing world.

I trust my inner guidance.

As I breathe into my body I feel trust, confidence,
and a secure sense of knowing deep within my core.

I have separated the next three conditions from the others. One, Alzheimer's, stands out for me because of the distinct stages of the disease. It is also not as common as the others. The second, obesity, is not yet classified as a disease, although it is certainly the cause of numerous diseases. And the third condition is a joyful one—pregnancy. I work with many couples who want to have a baby, and through the lens of energy medicine this process is awe-inspiring.

Alzheimer's

The *energetic intelligence* and physical process of Alzheimer's is slow and dramatic. I have watched my own father move through eleven years with this disease. One of many things that strike me about it is that the disease moves the person into three separate energetic states, all of which have different stages of awareness.

The first state is what I term the Zen Phase. Not everyone goes through this stage gently. My father was very contemplative. However, I know it was nothing short of devastating to him. What I mean by Zen is that due to the beginning of losing both short-term memory and cognitive function, in this energetic phase of Alzheimer's the person is confronted with "the now." He only has "this moment," which moves on to the next, then to the one after that, and on to another moment, ad infinitum. Each passing moment is cognitively released or pulled away from him into a void of non-thinking.

The second energetic state of awareness is what I call the Scrapbook Phase. You can sense and see snapshots of the person's life in the electromagnetic field. His entire field is filled with all of the past memories that are significant to him. These energetic scenes and pictures create a patchwork quilt or scrapbook look in the energy field. No matter where you turn your intuitive attention, you can feel and see these memories floating in the field. Familiar places show up in the pictures within the field. They can be very simple: his dinner chair, the view as he sits on the side of his bed, or the way the light switch looks. Or they can be very complex: dramatic memories of World

War II, or being five years old and looking down at the "miniature" cows while sitting in his father's lap flying in a 1920 airplane's open-air cockpit. The memories in this phase can also be philosophies, ideologies, or phrases in one's native or foreign language. For instance, my father is a Presbyterian minister, but Buddhist and Sanskrit chants just seem to pop out of nowhere; he smiles and then wonders where they came from. In short, memories from not only this life but the entire existence of the soul can bleed through the veils of consciousness.

These are all pictures that tell him he is safe. They gently move and rotate in and around the field, and when his conscious mind touches them they become alive within his mind. These pictures often become the redundant stories he tells and clings to over and over again. While still engaging in conversations with others, he associates his life with these snapshots of it. Some pictures can be happy, some sad, some can provoke anger. This phase, more than any other in any disease I have witnessed, reveals the true nature of the person's internal pictures. How does he view his life? Was it a fair one? Did he receive all that he needed? Did he accomplish his dreams and goals? Fortunately for my father and our family, he is a little Buddha.

Working with someone in the Scrapbook Phase carries a lot of spiritual power. It is typically the longest period of Alzheimer's. Any caretaker can compassionately guide the person to gently release the anger, or continue to express joy. You can even do this in silent prayer. Wherever he is, you love him, right there.

The third phase I term Spiritual Liberation. As the person moves from Scrapbook to Liberation, his spiritual energy starts to move inward, deep into the subconscious mind. This process reconnects him more seamlessly with his beautiful spiritual energy. He tends to energetically and spiritually move in and out of his body, not knowing where or with whom he is. In the latter stages of this phase he does not even know who he is. It can be difficult for loved ones to experience their once-vibrant family member in this phase. Difficult, yes, but it is important to know that he is making his way, very slowly, back home to Spirit. He will have full memory of his life, who he is, and who you are after he crosses. He has already chosen his favorite time frame to which he will return. This is often the case for people when they transition. For those with Alzheimer's it is most assuredly the case. I see this happening when people are in both the Scrapbook and Liberation phases. They choose their joyous moments to which they will return once they have released the body and crossed over to Spirit. Trust in the fact that their souls will always know your soul.

Now that I've gone over the phases, let us gain further understanding of the energetic structure of Alzheimer's. The energetic particles of this disease stay within close range of the physical body. They create an exchange, and flow from inside the head to the etheric field. The particles are soft, alternating in shape and size. They move at a slower pace except when the nervous system is heightened due to fear. When this occurs they move rapidly in chaotic patterns.

The third chakra, where one's personal sense of power is located, has also been saturated with these particles. This has an effect on the autonomic nervous system as a whole; however, the parasympathetic nervous system sustains more of the energetic patterning due to the continuous "flight or flight" experiences of anxiety that often accompany this condition. The particles can be intuitively seen moving up and down the back of the body around the spinal column, scattering when the energy field and nervous system are shocked by any perception or stimuli that is deemed threatening or unfamiliar. These soft, textured particles are light in color, white, gray, and bluish-gray, and fill the entire field with the progression of the disease, which gives a fog-like structure to the energy field during its early phases.

The cellular energetics of both the gray and white matter of the brain have an inward drawing motion. The affected cell's energy is markedly less vivid than that of healthy cells. Energetically, there is a damp and membranous light gray film that tends to cover the brain cells of the affected areas. This energetic film sweeps down over the head and the front of the face. Physically, it relates to the vacant look in the person's eyes. The densities of all of these energetic aspects worsen and become thicker as the condition progresses. Toward the final stages of this disease, the film has basically covered the entire energetic field. But this is not painful; it is the phase of Spiritual Liberation. The spirit is breaking free of the body.

Pictures of one's life fill the emotional field as the *emotional intelligence* copes with the memory-stripping nature of the disease. Again, this is most evident in the Scrapbook Phase. These pictures float gently in and out of the emotional energy field, never quite dissolving until the last stages of the condition. Components of the emotional intelligence and energy that accompany this condition include upward-thrusting energy due to overthinking; a strong, exacting mind stuck in overanalyzing; and retreating emotions. Much of the emotional intelligence of Alzheimer's resides within and stems from the third chakra. The liver, spleen, and stomach's energy tend to be overtaxed, as is the nervous system.

It takes a long time for chemistry, energy, and emotions to contribute to this or any disease state; by no means are they the sole cause. They are, however, layers of the parfait. Remove a layer of stress from one's early life and most conditions can often be avoided or diminished. We must always remember that we all die from something, an accident or a disease. Rarely do people just leave their bodies when they are done. There is usually a breakdown in the physical and energetic system in order for the Spirit to be released.

The *spiritual intelligence* is that of having access to the subconscious mind's power. The process of the disease takes people out of their cognitive, conscious minds and into their intuitive, subconscious minds. Their Spirits move in and out of their bodies during the middle and latter stages of Alzheimer's. It is through this spiritual movement that they gain more and more access to the other side and other dimensions of thought and reality. A sense of freedom is achieved through this process, and the gift is oftentimes presented to the caretakers and onlooking loved ones, as it is with many diseases. The loved ones watching can learn much.

The lessons learned with Alzheimer's are those of being unlimited and free. The soul takes this lesson with it as it leaves the body and ultimately finds freedom. When it wrestles with the condition in its earlier stages, the spiritual lessons are those of detachment. It is the ultimate process of letting go and being in the moment.

Please note that those with these conditions as well as caretakers and family members can use all of the following slogans. When the illness strikes, all are affected in some manner.

Balancing Slogans

My soul is at home in the healing light of God.

I am connected to God, my life, and my body.

I am at peace.

God is with me in every moment.

God and my soul are in charge.

As I breathe in I feel the infinite connection with God and my spirit.

Obesity

Obesity weighs heavily on the mind just as it does within the physical body. The energetic intelligence of obesity can be noted throughout the energy field and certainly within the fat cells of the body. The most prominent energetic quality in the electromagnetic field is that the normally brilliant light spectrum dulls. The light waves move more slowly and in longer patterns. More succinctly, when you are overweight your light does not shine as brightly due to the clouded, static energy surrounding the physical body. The colors are fully intact, but simply not as much light shines through. It could be compared to looking at the dulled light of the sun on a cloudy day compared to its brightness on a cloudless day. The intensity of light is much different.

In addition, any area of the body that holds extra weight, such as the upper or lower abdomen, hips, thighs, or arms, has a thicker density in the etheric field, the energy field closest to the physical body. If the person is healthy but overweight, this thicker field is clear or milky in color. If diseases or other conditions are starting to build, the darker particles begin to build as well and crystallize within the field.

If they are associated with loose, wiggly fat, the fat cells in the body have a damp heat to them. The emotions are of sadness, weeping, and depression. When fat is hard, so too are the energy grids around the cells. With hard fat the dampness and heat recede and become their opposite: cold and hard with emotions to match. Some people have a mixture. Intuitively connecting with the cells will tell you what and whose energy the person is holding. Sensitive people, empaths, and healthcare workers often hold fat on the body as a protection from other people's illnesses. Healthy personal values and boundaries keep most people's weight in check.

The *emotional intelligence* of obesity has a paradoxical nature. As I mentioned before, obese or overweight people tend to be sensitive as a whole. The less mature the person is in regard to their sensitivities, the greater the potential for weight gain. The two-year-old will come out and want what it wants. Often people are just oblivious to how energy affects them and how negative feelings cause them to be paralyzed (not exercise) and overeat (consume more calories than they expend). It is complicated and everyone is different, but there are common threads.

Sensitive people block unknown and unwelcome energy in a couple of ways. They disconnect from their bodies and operate only from the shoulders up. This disconnection allows them to move as quickly through their day as possible. They think they are in touch with their feelings, and in some ways they are. However, they are not in touch with what is happening below the neck, and their bodies pay the price. Others pull away from everyone and everything. Their entire bodies hide. So the energetic reverse of hiding happens. Hiding means covering up with pounds of protection. Women hide from men. Men hide from women. People hide from their gifts, various responsibilities, and the harder nature of what life offers at times.

Wanting love and acceptance from others is the primary emotional intelligence of being overweight. The antidote is self-love, taking back one's power, owning one's gifts, and developing stronger personal boundaries by taking responsibility for one's physical, emotional, and spiritual life. Love comes from others, yes; we all need and want that connection. You attract another's love equal to and based on the quality of love that is within you.

I don't dispute that eating calorie-laden foods filled with sugar, trans fats, and preservatives is toxic to most of the body's fat cells, but the electromagnetic field and the second and third chakras hold significant keys to unlocking obesity. They are the storytellers and provide the information needed to release the weight and let one's light shine. The second chakra governs sexual creative energy and the sense of taste. Is it any wonder that cravings for love, attention, peace and quiet, sovereignty, and money cause people to eat? That sense of taste has to be expressed and appeased somehow. There are many ways to use one's second-chakra energy; it is not all about food and sex. People who have lost weight and kept it off have turned things around in their second chakras. They have utilized their second-chakra energy in new and healthy patterns. They desire exercise, or at least they feel out of balance when they don't get it. They crave different tastes in food, those that keep their bodies healthy. If you have ever not eaten sugar for an extended period of time and then had some, you know the sweetness just about chokes you. Your tastes do change.

If you carry excess weight, tapping into your creative energy and putting it into right action can cure this condition. Cravings are an option in life; they are part of the continuum of desire for all of us. So what do you crave—success, love, carrots, exercise, chocolate? It is a matter of focus and choice. Always in the moment, you get to decide how to use your creative energy.

That choice is often dictated by the third chakra—your self-esteem, self-worth, and the conviction you hold for yourself. When your self-esteem is low, you know what happens. The bottom falls out of your life and your bottom may get bigger as a result. Only you can garner and harness your self-esteem. Following the intuitive impulse in the moment is a start. If it hits you to exercise, go! Don't sit there and let that "other" voice come in and say, "I will later." Later is in the future and never arrives.

The fear of rejection is the *spiritual intelligence* that creates the armor of obesity. There is also self-rejection that can happen at times before anyone else can reject you. Not everyone is going to agree with your worldview or even like you. If you are sensitive and intuitive, don't hide yourself because you're afraid that someone won't like or appreciate you. Don't believe that you will soak up all that fear and hold it in your body. Set up boundaries for yourself other than weight, and own your emotions with maturity. Don't waste your precious life energy positioning yourself to be okay for others. They aren't in your body. And if you happen to find someone else's energy in your body, do your electromagnetic field and fat cells a favor; get them out of there. Use the Running the Rainbow exercise, qigong, or tai chi to move energy, heal your body, and promote self-love. You can change your mind, change your energy, and change your body.

Embrace the fact that you have a right to be here. More importantly, your spirit has a mission on earth within this lifetime. You have the obligation to engage in that mission. Use your second-chakra energy to ignite a new vision for yourself. Take small steps and move in that direction every day. With each decision you get closer to your arrival. Make good choices that are founded on the spiritual lesson that is so prevalent with obesity—self-love. What will you do today to allow yourself to feel love and connection? It does not have to involve anyone else. You are all you have anyway; everything and everyone else in your life is an extra treat and connection. Your connection to yourself is the spiritual goal of this lesson.

Balancing Slogans

I am connected to my body and its needs.

I have respect for my precious life.

I love my life.

I know who I am.

I know what's good for me.

With every breath I take I feel connected to my body.

I know and understand my life's work and joyfully pursue it every day.

I am here to live fully and be a blessing to this earth.

Pregnancy

One of the most rewarding aspects of my work is to receive pictures of little ones who have come into this world. It is a miracle to be a witness to how Spirit works. I am inspired when I see a future baby in the mother's energy field weeks, months, and in some cases, years before her conception and birth.

The *energetic intelligence* of pregnancy is such that the spirit of the unborn child moves into the energy field of the mother prior to conception. Energetically, her structure is about the size of a golf ball, at times a bit larger. The colors in this small orb consist of lights so brilliant that a Crayola sixty-four-pack could only hope to combine colors to match this vibrant perfection.

One day I was driving down the road and my sister-in-law popped into my mind. I saw the shimmering little light of my nephew, and knew he was on the way. He was hovering slightly left of her left hip. Suddenly, this little light zoomed into her body. I called her that evening and asked if there was anything new or anything she wanted to tell me. She told me that the strangest feeling had come over her that she was pregnant. She took a test a week or two later and, sure enough, a son was on the way.

The *emotional* and *spiritual intelligences* of pregnancy are very tightly woven together, so I have combined them. The energy of the woman's body needs to be in balanced shape for most pregnancies to occur. However, if those babies want to come in, they will come in, no matter what. In my experience, in order for a conception to take place and a pregnancy to hold there has to be agreement on both sides: the parents, mostly the mother, and the spirit of the child-to-be. When there is a miscarriage, there is not an agreement to hold the pregnancy on a spiritual level; other lessons are embedded within these experiences.

While the pregnant mother waits and nurtures her unborn child, the spiritual intelligence and emotional energy of pregnancy become very prominent. The energy of the child's Spirit moves in and out of the mother's body. It does so in preparation for birth. It is gathering energy, instructions, and lessons to be learned. It is gaining the spiritual energy, or the consciousness, that it will carry forth through its lifetime. Shortly before birth, all of this spiritual intelligence sinks into the subconscious mind to be brought to the surface later through life's occurrences.

Many women can feel or sense their child moving in or out of their bodies. Even when the baby is in the last trimester and is kicking and hiccupping, they can feel the Spirit of the child moving in and around them. The mother and the child's Spirit are joined by loving relatives who have crossed over to the other side and are helping the Spirit of the child prepare. Angels, guides, and support from the Spiritual World are all there. They love, teach, guide, and protect the Spirit of the unborn child. I have yet to see any child come into this world without the help of those who will walk with them in spirit as the child grows and lives his human life.

Personality characteristics, musical gifts, scholarly aptitudes, and some of what the child will both give and receive from his forthcoming physical life are all present within the energy that is this little ball of light reflecting the massive energy of the Spirit. Not everything is revealed about the life of the child; that would leave no surprises, and the lessons that will guide the child and family through their human journey would thereby be denied. We don't have *that* much control over things—even though we'd like to think we do.

You cannot force a child to come into this world. But whether you are destined to have children through natural birth, medically supported conceptions, or adoption, your dreams of parenthood will come true. Destiny can only be walked with, never pushed away, rushed, or coerced.

If you want to become pregnant, follow your inner guidance. Seek appropriate health care. Provide your body with excellent nutrition before becoming pregnant if possible. Traditional Chinese medicine, especially acupuncture, can be very helpful. Also, practices such as yoga and meditation are excellent for keeping yourself healthy and energetically and spiritually balanced.

Balancing Slogan:

I openly and joyfully receive this child.

As I breathe deeply into my body I feel health, openness, and energy.

*I am ready to love this child and supply inspiration
for its life's journey.*

8

Creating Intuitive Wellness

Every day you get the chance to trust yourself more.

We are here for only a short while. The months and years of a lifetime whisk by and we wonder where it has all gone. That is why we must enjoy and embrace life as robustly as we possibly can. We will all arrive at the time when we are close to death, then taste the sweetness of holy light pouring over us from a place beyond the physical. No matter what our age, a storm can figuratively or literally blast into our life without warning; everything can be transformed or lost within minutes. We should therefore embrace life gently and fully, creating wellness in every moment.

In that spirit, I offer in this chapter concepts for your daily contemplation that will assist you in creating, supporting, and maintaining your intuitive wellness. Intuitive wellness is wellness in all areas of your life, based on the knowledge you derive from your inner well of wisdom. Go into the silence of yourself daily and ask for the intuitive guidance you need to create and support your wellness that day. Then practice the art of implementing the wisdom that you have received.

Practice Detachment

A wonderful movie called *Auntie Mame* has one of my favorite lines: "Life is a banquet, and most poor suckers are starving to death." Life is full of experiences that can remind us to let go of the things keeping us from the banquet table and more fully embrace the love of God. I urge you to let go of the things to which you cling. If you are meant to have something or someone in your life, they will not leave you. People, objects, and situations are woven like the threads of a fabric; the nature of the weaving will determine whether it holds or not. You can mend and patch, but if a tear is meant to be, it will happen. So be at peace with the way people and objects weave through your life.

I am not suggesting that you have to give away all that you have accumulated. But what you are attached to will leave you at some point. When a strong attachment to a person, object, or belief exits your life, you will experience suffering, which is only a natural process of the mind and heart. Through the use of your mind and intuition, you can ease that suffering by realizing that your mind is the source of your thoughts—thoughts that can spin into attachment and suffering. You can, therefore, use that same mind to shift your thoughts, change the way you perceive relationships, objects, and experiences, and get on the pathway to peace. Use your intuition to see and know what the truth is.

When people practice detachment, they report feeling more joy, freedom, and balance. That's because with greater detachment, you create the space for life's synchronicities to enter your journey and more fully tune in to your innate wisdom. When you are less attached to doing things a certain way or having certain things and people around, you will more easily hear your inner voice directing you. Listen deeply to that voice every day. Do not pass by life's banquet table, which is filled with the delicious sustenance of God.

Daily Intuitive Wellness

Enlightenment is achieved by working in a disciplined manner on your spirit-led path. This is not an easy task, but it is an important one, because your daily spiritual practice is your connection to what is true about your life. The truth that comes from the innate wisdom deep within you is the centering device that will assist you in maintaining balance in your being. I have heard it said, "Enlightenment is easy, keeping it is difficult."

To find wisdom and wellness, close your eyes and, with your intuitive mind, read from the book of your soul. The truth and answers you seek will come forth through the thought forms that reside in your atomic structure. Whether you are peering into the atomic structure of your energy or your body, you will find that truth and wisdom reside in these particles of thought. Truth and wisdom cannot be joined with your bodily senses or intelligence unless those senses— smell, sight, hearing, taste, and touch—are joined first with your intuition. There is, of course, wisdom in the sensations of the body and mind, but to reach the depth that is God-realized, your search needs to be intuitively guided into the infinitesimal parts of yourself and your atomic and subatomic energy. To accomplish this journey you need to practice daily.

For daily intuitive wellness, I suggest you set aside anywhere from twenty minutes to an hour, one or two times per day, to work with whatever exercises in this book speak to you, or any other practices you feel drawn to, such as meditation, chanting, tai chi, or walking in nature. Although there are many types of religious institutions in

Western culture, some people feel spiritually empty and unfulfilled. It is important to have a spiritual path as you move forward. The path need not be a traditional religion. What really matters is that your spirit feels well on your chosen path; if it doesn't feel right deep down inside, commit to your wisdom and search for the path that is best for you.

In order to successfully develop your intuition for daily wellness and abundance, give your practice and intention priority in your daily schedule. In your busy life, it may be easy to push inner work aside, leaving it to collect dust. However, the dust is really collecting inside you, shutting you off from realizing your desires for happiness and an end to suffering. There is always a place or time in which you can go within and find inner peace. I have a friend who meditates on the subway from her Manhattan office to her Brooklyn home. Wherever you are, your inner self is with you.

Spiritual Teachers

Life and its experiences of each moment are your teachers. And the best teacher is the one within. However, on your spiritual path you may feel that you would benefit from a teacher or mentor. By all means, seek out a spiritual teacher if you are called to do so. A teacher should demonstrate what you wish to become, and understand that what you seek is already within you. I'd like to share what I've learned about seeking outside guidance and working with spiritual teachers.

Start by having a sense of what a teacher should be like for you. A spiritual teacher's desire is to guide you toward your awakening. As you begin to awaken to your own innate wisdom, divisions between you and your teacher will diminish. You will become as one. All the masters report this. Christ shared this view. The Buddha spoke of it as well. The role of the teacher is to show that the student who loves, believes, and is dedicated to the wisdom of Spirit, God, and Oneness, as the teacher demonstrates, will be able to perform deeds as great as the teacher can. Entire philosophies are based on this and other supportive precepts. Spiritual teachings are also a matter of vibration. A teacher cannot teach anyone who vibrates higher than the teacher himself. Seek a teacher or spiritual essence that is like that of the moon, not the finger pointing at the moon.

You should not feel engulfed by your teacher. If you do feel consumed, talk to your body, mind, and spirit and commit to your own non-ego-based wisdom. In other words, be honest with yourself regarding the situation. A teacher will, while embracing and supporting you, also demand that you pull your own spiritual weight. Such insistence will allow you to find your own true nature, which is the nature of God. As this process unfolds, differences between you and your teacher, as well as the apparent divisions between darkness and enlightenment, will soften and fade.

A spiritual teacher will assist you in stretching your consciousness, which may not be easy or comfortable at the time. Nonetheless, your teacher will push you with love because he or she can see the levels of consciousness you are here to work on—and can reach. A teacher desires nothing more than for you to achieve peace and enlightenment for yourself and your soul.

It is up to you to choose your spiritual teacher wisely. Be certain that you are ready to commit to your wisdom and learn from your teacher's wisdom. Know that, as with other things or people in your life, you may not need to be under your chosen teacher's wings for a long period of time. Develop your own sense of intuition so that you are clear inside about which teacher you should work with, and for how long. I have seen people who have no third-chakra energy of their own attach themselves to a teacher or teaching. They lose their sense of self while claiming devotion; but devotion is a process of the heart chakra, not the third chakra. Your path is best served by loving kindness and balance.

As you show love, respect, compassion, and honor for your teacher, you will receive them in kind. A teacher will empower and assist you in realizing your God-given wisdom and strength, and encourage you to share what you have learned with others, in your own way and using your own nature. A teacher may not give you everything you ask for or expect regarding your work and growth. A wise teacher will know exactly where you are and what you need at that point. Your journey will be less difficult if you accept that and know that your teacher will lead you as best fits you, however difficult it might seem at times.

When the right teacher arrives, be grateful. Participate as fully as you can, using your innate wisdom and your faculties of reason to discern both the teacher and the teachings. Be willing to share knowledge with others, and understand that when someone offers you advice, whether you take it or not, they are demonstrating that they are your teacher. Make note of their acts of kindness and sharing. Be a disciple, whatever you do and with whomever you come in contact. You never know who is a Buddha or angel in disguise. Keep in mind these Buddhist sutras (the Buddha's teachings given orally to his disciples and then later put into written form):

Do not rely on the individual teachers; rely on the teachings.

Do not rely on the words; rely on the meanings.

Do not rely on the adapted or conventional meaning; rely on the ultimate, absolute meaning.

Do not rely on intellectual knowledge; rely on wisdom.

Know that your greatest teachers will be the discoveries that lead to what innately lies inside you. Be thankful for the blessing of being alive and having the power of mind and truth of heart to change your world and help others do the same.

Knowing Your Truths

Knowing your inner truths is key to attaining and nurturing intuitive wellness. If you are not following some of your truths, you may not feel as well as you could. Since you know what you want out of your life, you most likely understand the underlying truths that support you on your journey. It is imperative to know them, see them daily, and embrace them always.

Here is a simple exercise I would like you to play with. It has been helpful for me and has assisted many others in examining their beliefs. Take a look at the following list of personal truths. These are my truths, reflections of my teacher within. I suggest that you too make a list of your truths. You can write them down and tape the list to your desk or make a screen saver out of them. You can look at them when you are not flowing through your day as you'd like to. The truths you are not following closely will light up for you, create pause and realignment, and reestablish a sense of inner peace.

Trust and commit to my wisdom
Mindfully live in the moment
Honor myself daily
Listen to the birds
Watch the clouds
Remember the bigger picture of life as I
move through daily situations
Remember my purpose and my work
Endeavor to bring peace within and without
Sing

Feel compassion for all beings
Be loving kindness
Go into the silence daily
Listen
Jump for joy
Stand up for my rights, feelings, and purpose
Share with others
Live simply
Serve others
Have fun
Hug trees
Be in awe of the sky and land around me
Honor animals without hips and shoulders
Move my body daily
Eat in a sacred way
Keep in contact with those I love
Be honest with myself and others
Live happily
Listen to the clue of sadness
Honor my emotions and my mind
Write
Obtain and share knowledge
Listen to my guidance
Discern
Honor ceremony
Always set a sacred space for myself
Honor the paradoxes in life
Be free
Share love
Keep on
Dig deep

Reach high
Think unlimited thoughts in directions that move me
Go for it
Spread joy
Stay humble but not quiet
Roar
Weep
Stay on my path but know that forks exist
Glow
Get into the energy of life
Always practice attentiveness of mind
Be generous

Keep Evolving

Make an effort to be happy in your daily practice and life, releasing negative thoughts as they arise in your mind. Practice the virtuous actions of loving kindness, generosity, patience, discipline, and effort. Whenever a negative or unsettling thought arises, engage your spiritual practice (a practice that you never, in fact, leave). Bring forth from your mind an antidote for your anger or unsettledness; the exercises in this book will help with this. Feelings of compassion and joy are also antidotes. Wash your mind with compassion and know that the negative feelings will hold no strength over you. When you are feeling negative emotions, feel compassion for yourself.

Over the course of many lifetimes and life experiences, you have created the karma and the wisdom that are currently within you. They dictate the levels of consciousness you are able to perceive and, consequently, your ability to work through the phenomena associated with those particular levels of consciousness. Each time you arrest the negative emotions that arise in your mind, replacing them with thoughts and positive actions, actions that benefit others, you gain more of the pure cosmic mind, the mind of God.

There is a circle of people you will touch during this lifetime. You are their guardian, as they are yours. The experience of near death and joining with others' souls, along with other experiences in my life, have demonstrated to me that we don't die. Our souls live on, growing and evolving. The more we can consciously tap into our soul-level existence and anchor that connection within our physical body, the more virtuous actions we can bring forth. The desires to have and hold objects or people in our reality fade as our awareness of impermanence, along with the knowledge of our eternal souls, increases. These are all gained through practice.

Your eternal soul flows like a river throughout eternity. When left unrestrained, it will follow its own natural impulses, drifting and rushing toward the ocean of wisdom, the one true source. Do not restrict your consciousness with negative thoughts or emotions, or you will stagnate. Allow the pure, living waters of your soul and consciousness to refresh yourself and others. Allow your soul, mind, and body to flow into wellness, enlightenment, and peace.

Within these pages I have offered my knowledge of intuition and my personal journey so you will have the principles and the practical application for creating your own intuitive wellness. As I wrote in the preface, my wish is to give you the wings to fly toward wellness and enlightenment. I have always believed that intuition is a divine skill we all have inside us; it is simply a matter of trusting the wisdom within and allowing it to lead us to untold levels of peace and healing. The rewards, as you will see, are limitless: hearing your body's messages, sensing the energy moving through your personal energy system, resolving emotional and physical pain, and developing trust and confidence in your own innate wisdom. Inner healing is indeed within your grasp, and the time to embrace it is now.

Appendix
Exercises to Clear the Mind, Nurture the Body, and Create Wellness

Creating Sacred Space

The environment in which you meditate, visualize, and pray plays an important part in the effectiveness of your spiritual practice. As your intuition and spiritual nature develop and season, you will be able to stay calm and centered even in the most distracting situations and environments. It is best to have a sacred space in your own home in which to practice. Creating this type of space in your home will lead to a calmness and centeredness in your being and your life.

Your sacred space does not have to consist of an entire room or wing of the house; it can simply be a tabletop in your favorite room. Creating sacred space in your bedroom is always nice because as you enter sleep and the dream state at night you will already have a wonderful energy of consciousness in place surrounding you. Your consciousness is highly suggestible when you are in the sleep state, so why not be the one who creates the space in which your consciousness rests?

If you are really cramped for space, or whoever you live with doesn't understand your spiritual quest, you don't need a permanent sacred place. What truly matters is what resides in your own heart space.

If your space is limited, if you have other constraints, or if you travel often, you can create a portable altar. Simply take a small piece of cloth—a foot square works well—and set your sacred items on top of it to create a spiritual space. When you are not engaged in a sacred practice of some kind, you can simply wrap up your items and store them in the cloth. Place the bundle in a dresser drawer or a box when not in use. When you are ready to meditate, pray, or do whatever practice you use to enhance your spiritual growth, place your altar items reverently on the cloth before you begin. When you are finished, give thanks, gently wrap them back up in the cloth, and put them away.

What things might you put on your altar? A good foundation is important, so it is nice to have a decorative piece of fabric or cloth upon which to set your items. It is preferable to select something made of a natural or organic fabric such as cotton or silk. Natural fabrics conduct energy differently from fabrics such as rayon, polyester, or synthetic blends. Natural is natural, and that is what you want to connect with, your natural energy. To support that process with the natural items on your altar only makes sense. This type of cloth is easily available and comes in a wide variety of colors and patterns.

Items that you set upon your altar should have significance for you; they need to touch your soul. You might have a bouquet of fresh flowers, or, if space is limited, even a single flower. Items such as rocks, crystals, fossils, or feathers that you have found or purchased from an interesting place add grounded earth energy.

You may choose to place on your altar a picture of a loved one or an exalted master who touches you. Pictures of masters such as Jesus, Mary, Buddha, Hindu gods or goddesses, saints from any religion, a

cherished guru (teacher), or pictures of indigenous guides and symbols are all appropriate. After all, this is your sacred space and your
altar should bring to it the energies and levels of consciousness that
are meaningful to you. Furthermore, having such masters present will
assist you in keeping focused on whatever level of consciousness you
would like to resonate with and therefore achieve.

Your sacred space will most likely change as you change. As your
spirit grows and soars, the way you express your spirit and spirituality will change accordingly. All things are impermanent. Think of
the beautiful and meaningful sand paintings of the Native Americans
or the colorful sand mandalas of the Tibetan Buddhists. They are
sacred spaces filled with holy artistic meanings, created to evoke energies and certain levels of consciousness for particular events. These
beautiful creations are used for worship in their cultural context
and then destroyed, releasing the spirit and displaying a nonattach-
ment to form.

Use your sacred space whenever your schedule allows. Optimally,
it is beneficial to sit quietly in this space and practice mediation, do
some journaling, read spiritually comforting and expanding books,
or experience some of the exercises in this book. You will find it
helpful to do this at least once a day, even if it is only for ten to fifteen minutes. The best times to use this space for practice are in the
early morning and right before you go to bed. Obviously, the more
time you devote to your practices, the more benefit you will
receive. Any time is a good time to go inward and experience the
sweet depth of yourself.

Introduction to Your Soul

This visualization will introduce you to something you may not have
seen or connected with in a long time, if ever: your soul. After engaging

in this quick, simple exercise, you may wonder why it has taken so long to view this wondrous part of yourself!

Visualization is the process of creating mental images with your mind. You are visualizing or imagining things that you want to bring into your life. You can visualize a healthy body, a rewarding relationship, or a more abundant lifestyle; what you put your efforts toward will come to pass. When you access your intuition and intend to call forth a spiritually profound aspect of yourself, you may be surprised at the visualization that enters your mind. It could be very different from what you could have imagined just by holding a thought of an object or something desired with your mind. Merging an intuitively driven intention with the power of visualization creates a powerful presence within you, a presence that truly captures the spiritual essence of who you are.

It is best to do this exercise in a peaceful space. If you have already gathered materials for your altar and created a sacred space, invoke the sacredness of the space and allow it to engulf you. You may choose to play some soft, soothing music in the background. Next, sit comfortably, upright in a chair, gather your thoughts inward, and let go of the outside world. Now ask that an image of your soul be presented to you. You may see an image that looks similar to a human form. Or you may see sparks of light or larger balls of light. Set the intention and hold your attention clearly so that you can be introduced to your own magnificence.

Sit quietly while the image (or images) appears. Trust your intuitive wisdom; don't sweep away any images in disbelief. Listen to, see, feel, and know your spiritual truth. You are asking to see who you are, your true self: an awesome gift and experience.

Once you have the image in front of you, ask any question you desire. If you have been struggling with a certain problem—physical or emotional—now is the time to ask for assistance. Listen and take in any information that may be given to you. When you are finished receiving the insights that your soul's image has for you, invite it to join you in your physical body, integrating your soul's energy with your physical being. This is accomplished by seeing, feeling, or knowing that this energetic form of your soul is gently and safely merging with your body. If the image is in a humanlike or angelic form, watch as it sits inside your body; allow it to slide into your body like a hand into a glove. If the image is a spark, ball of light, or anything else, permit it to merge with your body in the way in which you are directed. I can tell you from my experience and that of others that when you join with soul-level energy, wondrous things appear, challenges diminish, and peace begins to bathe you.

If there is any hesitation on your part to invite this soulful energy and consciousness inside your physical form, trust that knowledge as well. This initial time may not be the one in which you are to merge. Simply move at your pace, in accordance with your guidance. You are in control of this visualization.

I suggest you do this exercise whenever you are drawn to it, especially if you are feeling disconnected or confused about who you are and what your purpose is. It will offer you some peace of mind as it brings into your conscious awareness the eternal connection that is ever-present.

Intuitive Shopping

Go through the grocery store while tuning in to your intuition. Choose your food from that perspective. Literally stand in the produce section, for instance, and see which fruits or vegetables speak to you through your senses. Tune in and listen to the ones that call you. Or feel, with intuitive hands, which ones want to go home with you and nourish your body. Pay attention to the smells that appeal to you. If you regularly choose your food in this way, your eating cannot help but change for the better: You will feel the difference between those foods in the produce section and, say, the chip and soda pop aisle. You will be able to discern the difference between the energies and consciousnesses of the fresher, organic foods and the more heavily processed ones. Rest assured that your body can tell the difference. We have been so programmed by the media and society regarding what to eat that we forget to listen to our body's wisdom as to what it needs. Begin to listen again. Your intuition can guide you in everything you do, every step of the way. Your task is to simply listen, pay attention, and commit to your intuitive wisdom in a trusting way, moment to moment.

Releasing Mind Chatter

Here is a simple way to release mind chatter. You can do this practice alone or with a partner. Take ten minutes out of your day and sit and just let your thoughts roll from your mind and out of your mouth. Whatever thought comes to your mind, speak it. Let the thought that sits behind or connects to the previous thought rise up and be spoken also. One after another the thoughts will come rolling off your tongue. It doesn't matter if they seem connected or not; just let them roll—no judgment, no self-counseling (if you are doing this by yourself), no fixing, or stopping—just let go of your thoughts. The power of release comes in the vocalization of the thoughts, so speak them boldly. Lift up your voice, intone, and release your emotions. Let your thoughts and voice join to let go of the chattering that fills your mind. After this practice, you'll feel relieved and refreshed. Do it regularly to avoid mental buildup.

If you choose to do the exercise with a partner, follow the directions above, but sit facing in opposite directions with your right shoulder slightly touching your partner's right shoulder. The purpose behind this arrangement is to allow no space for judgment, consoling, fixing, or pampering. The benefit to the speaker is to have a silent, non-judgmental witness. We rarely do that for ourselves—refrain from judging. It is an interesting experience to have another person hold that type of space open for us. Do the exercise without any eye contact or other physical contact that could distract the speaker. And because you and your partner are facing in opposite directions, none of the vocalized energy from one person will get on or attach to the other.

This is an especially powerful tool in a partnership situation; it is intimate, supportive, nonjudgmental, and freeing. Last, understand that when you are finished speaking, you are finished. There is no going back and discussing what was said. It's over. Do not attach or hang onto anything that was said. You can do this practice in as little as ten minutes per speaker, or for up to thirty minutes. It all depends on how much time you have and how much chatter you need to let go of.

Calming the Mind Through Breath

Breathing is one of your body's involuntary functions. If you are alive, your body is doing it, whether or not you think about it. Nonetheless, you can also control the breath to some extent. Exercises in breath control, such as breath retention and deliberate methods of inhalation and exhalation, are used for specific mental and physical benefits. These exercises are called Pranayama.

The techniques of Pranayama come to us through the path of yoga. *Prana* means life force and *ayama* means to control or master. The style of pranayama breathing that I teach my clients and students and am sharing with you is called Ujjaya (OOO-ji-ya). It is also referred to as Ocean Breath, Hissing Breath, Victorious Breath, and Darth Vader Breath (referring to the movie *StarWars*).

When you practice Ujjaya Breath you will calm your mind, enhance your attention span and mental capacity, bring more oxygen into the body, and stimulate your circulation and metabolism. This breath induces a calm meditative state, as your mind is gently absorbed into the sound of the breath. To do this breath, you will slightly contract the glottis in the back of your throat while you inhale and exhale. It may feel and sound as if you are softly snoring.

1. Sit in a comfortable position with your spine erect, or you can lie down on your back.

2. Begin by taking slow, deep breaths in through your nostrils. Exhale through your mouth. Allow the breath to be gentle and relaxed.

3. Now slightly contract the back of your throat near the glottis, creating a steady, raspy sound as you breathe in and out. The sound need not be forced and it should only be loud enough that someone near you could hear it. You can keep your mouth open or closed as you prefer.

4. Lengthen the exhalations and inhalations as much as possible without creating any tension anywhere else in your body. Allow the sound of the breath to be continuous and smooth, like rolling ocean waves. For a more advanced practice, allow the connection between the inhalation and exhalation to be as seamless as possible.

Running the Rainbow

This is a popular exercise with my clients, one that they return to often in their daily practices. Running the Rainbow is an extraordinarily powerful way to clear unwanted energetic debris and influences from your energy field, and ultimately your physical body. Even if you do it just once, I believe you'll be moved. Done regularly over time, it is an excellent tool that allows you to become more aware of the way energy moves through your body.

It is especially important to record your experience in your journal each time you do this exercise. Writing down your experience is necessary to work through what I call "energy mapping." Mapping is the process by which you uncover submerged patterns of energy, emotions, thought forms, and behaviors. The process involves writing down your experience as though you were simply the observer and therefore objectively reporting how the colors move through your body. As you work with this exercise over a period of time, patterns in the way your energy flows will begin to emerge. This mapping will give you information about the most effective way you can utilize your life-force energy. If you do the exercise once a day for, say, thirty days, you will begin to be able to discern much more clearly what serves you in your life and what doesn't.

You might wonder how this happens. During the process of Running the Rainbow, you are bringing into your body the colors of the rainbow—red, orange, yellow, green, blue, indigo, and violet—through the physical and energetic layers that invisibly surround your physical body. We know scientifically that colors have and hold vibrational rates within their molecular structure that are specific to each color band. We also know that each of your bones and muscle tissues, as well as your vital organs and all other bodily components, has and holds a specific vibrational rate that is relative to it.

When you run the colors of the rainbow one by one through your body, the color's vibrational rates will affect your body's vibrational rates, both overall and within each individual section of the body. In addition, any person's or place's energy that may have temporarily taken up residence somewhere in your body's energetic field will be affected by a color's vibrational rate as it passes through your systems, causing changes, albeit subtle ones in the beginning.

The river of life-force energy that moves through you and on to others encompasses all the colors of the rainbow. At times, some colors are more prevalent in the electromagnetic field than others, and this is often due to your current state of wellness—in other words, how you're feeling about yourself and your world, mentally, physically, emotionally, and spiritually. In addition, the various energies and levels of consciousness that are flowing in and out of your life and your body appear as colored bands and currents of energy in the electromagnetic field.

Begin by grounding yourself. This is done simply by using your mind's eye (the sixth chakra) to imagine cords or roots extending from the soles (souls) of your feet and sinking deep into the earth; see them deeply penetrating through the earth's crust. Let this grounded feeling spread throughout your body. Sense the energy of the earth and your connection to it. Know that you are safe and secure and working with your body's energy.

Now visualize the following colors rising up one by one through the grounding cords or roots. Work with the colors in order at first; then, after you've gained some experience, trust your intuitive wisdom as to the sequence of color appropriate for you. The order of the colors is as follows: red—first chakra; orange—second chakra; yellow—third chakra; green—fourth chakra; sky blue—fifth chakra; indigo—sixth chakra; violet—seventh chakra. Run each color individually up through the grounding cords connected to your feet and to the top of your head. Then allow the color to branch at the throat and cascade down your arms, flowing out the palms of your hands.

Now comes the actual energy mapping. As you run your rainbow, holding your mind in the place of observer, examine how each color feels while it's in your body. Is it warm, hot, cool, or cold? Pay attention to the color's viscosity; is it thick or thin? Notice the texture of the color, of the energy (if there is any), as well as the way the color flows through your body—with how much ease or difficulty.

Notice any images that pop into your mind as you run a particular color. Does a person or event you haven't thought of for awhile come to mind? Do any emotions rise within you? Pay attention to every detail; play with the image; relax and trust yourself. Just let things happen.

Change from one chakra color to the next by replacing the color with the next color in line. For example, to transition from red (first chakra) to orange (second chakra), simply allow the red color to continue flowing out the top of your head and the palms of your hands while the new color, in this case orange, begins to flow up through the grounding cords and into your body. Run each color through your body as long as you like; you'll know when it's time to switch colors.

Some people find it difficult to run colors from their feet upward, and yet find it easy to run the colors down from the top of the head and body, and then ground them into the earth. It is fine if you choose to do it that way; it simply allows for a different perspective. However, the reason I suggest that you run your rainbow from the ground up is that it will ground you in your body.

Work with this exercise for at least thirty days in a row and your intuitive abilities will become more apparent. You will recognize that you already know what is best for you, your body, and your energy.

Dealing with Blockages

When you work with the Running the Rainbow exercise or other exercises in this book, you will undoubtedly find places in your body and its energy system that have resistance or blockages. At times, a blockage you discover could have been there for decades. You don't necessarily want to focus on getting it out of you. Once you find a little or big blockage, you have to be brave enough to mindfully dive into the middle of the mess and see what's up. Don't panic. It's you in there, at least a part of you. You may not like it, but it's all you.

You will find that asking questions is a vital part of clearing blockages, and of intuitive work in general. As you learn to work with your intuition, your body, and its energies, you will also learn how best to ask the questions. Your questions will likely be framed around who, what, when, and where. I suggest that you don't focus on "why" too much. For one thing, it doesn't solve the issue; for another, it's more like whining to the universe. Personally, I use the word "what" a lot when I ask questions. That word will give you more intuitive direction when dealing with your blockages. It will also guide you more clearly toward the antidote for your issue.

The following exercise contains ideas for questions that can uncover a blockage. Use it to mindfully access, identify, and transform any issue that is blocking your personal energy system.

1. Begin by taking a few cleansing breaths into your body. Connect with your body and ask, yes ask, to be made aware of any blockages that you are currently experiencing. Listen to what your body says, the direction your attention is drawn to, or any visual picture you receive in your mind's eye. Trust whatever answer you intuitively receive.

Once you locate the initial blockage, you must ask that part of your body if there is any energy extending from that blockage that also connects to another place, chakra, or organ system within your body. Like a plant's roots, energy blockages can send out shoots of energy and spread negative thoughts, behaviors, and emotions into other areas. You want to make certain that when you go in to work with one of your blockages, you have access to all its offshoots. Fear can spawn its cousins: anger, distrust, and sadness. Be attentive and gentle, and awaken to who and what is rooting itself in your chakra.

2. Ask the energies what primary emotions are associated with this blockage; is there anger, fear, distrust, or envy? Make note of what you intuitively hear, see, feel, or know.

3. Ask those emotions what opposite thought would be their antidote. Everything has a voice, and as you use your intuition, it will tell you.

For example, you have found a block in your third chakra with tangents into the second chakra. The blockage could appear this way: The energy in your third chakra is darker and harder in one area. You sense a compaction of emotions such as sadness, anger, or concern. You also notice that filaments of light extend down into the second chakra. The colors in these filaments are slightly different from the dark colors of the initial block, but they have similar characteristics. The texture is the same, the colors are of the same hue, and the emotions are similar as well. You sense that the emotion around the blockage is fear. Further, it is draining your creative energy by sustaining behaviors of avoidance. If you have ever been afraid to do something, you know it takes more energy to avoid it than to accomplish it.

When you find a bundle of negative energy such as this, ask it what it needs. Mindfully await your answer. You hear from your body's energy that you are afraid to be rejected, so you don't extend yourself to others. You avoid living a full and productive life.

Now there are a lot of questions you could ask this energy. You can ask, *When did this start? What am I to learn from this? Where else in my body or life is this energy?* Some of the most important questions to ask are, *What can correct this? What is the antidote, in the form of the opposite thought, which will create balance in this energy?* For instance, if the emotion and thought are about fear, the body could respond by saying, *It is peace and confidence that I want.*

4. Ask your body what color(s) exemplify the new antidote thought. In the case of our example, your body may respond by saying, *Pink and blue are the colors that mirror peace and confidence.* To accelerate the healing you can breathe the colors pink and blue into the blockage.

5. Once you find out this information, sit comfortably and imagine that you are planting this new seed thought by breathing the colors and words deeply into that specific location in your body. So in our example, you breathe in the colors pink and blue, and plant the seed thoughts of *peace* and *confidence*. You are replacing the thoughts of fear and whatever grows from that. Continue this breathing pattern and thoughtful meditation for as long as you like. Your body will tell you when it feels complete with the process. You will simply know. And that, in and of itself, is a skill you are building: trusting and knowing what you need, when, where, how much, and for how long.

While breathing in pink and blue or any other color will not solely cure your cancer or stop a messy marriage from being a disaster, it can bring out stages of healing that are truly palpable and beneficial. Colors stimulate our nervous system and emotions. Color is a powerful representative of consciousness and is used as a descriptor of mood: feeling *blue*, so angry they see *red*. This is why we use color in our visualizations of healing. When your body has a blockage of anger or sadness there will be specific colors that reflect those emotions. You will want to ask your body to tell you the antidote for those negative feelings. When you visualize those colors within your body, they vibrate and represent the consciousness of calmness or peace. That's a process of healing.

In addition to the calming effects of breath, planting new seed thoughts creates different chemistry potentials. We know that habitual thoughts and behaviors have specific neuropathways in the brain. When you consciously and consistently focus on a thought, your brain supports existing neuropathways or creates new ones and releases the appropriate neurotransmitters. This is what Dr. Candice Pert refers to as *the molecules of emotions*. These positive thoughts stimulate the same pathways and chemistry and become physical habits; your way of being transforms and conforms.

Don't expect to heal twenty years of suffering in a few moments. However, I will tell you that many of my clients say they experience a difference in their bodies and emotions almost instantly. They feel calmer and more peaceful right away, which creates space for more healing to come. They go back to this simple exercise over and over again, and over time, they are no longer bothered by old behaviors that had sabotaged their lives in the past. Always remember that emotions stimulate your body to release chemicals. Ask yourself whether it would be more healing for you to have the emotions of peace and confidence stimulating your body's chemistry, or thoughts of fear and anger. You may chuckle at the obvious answer, but I ask, What are you doing about it? It's your body. It's your life. You are in charge.

Connecting with the Earth

Some of you are pent up in offices, grinding your way to and from work. Some of you are in a constant state of what I call "travel aerobics."

You dash from city to city, country to country via any mode of transportation that can get you there, and preferably on time. Even if you work in your home, which at times can be even more confining, you've got to get out and just walk the earth.

One of the major issues that contributes to stress overload, which in turn contributes to depression and anxiety, is that we do not connect with the earth. We are industrial as a culture. No longer do we fit the agrarian or horticultural patterns of society. Within those past social structures we depended on the earth for our daily existence and sustenance. We now build "things" that withstand the seasonal weather patterns that used to force migration. Technology is not a bad thing, but it does remove us from the earth as the dynamic force in our lives. I feel that this disconnect hinders our creative imaginations and deadens our intuitive natures.

Most people understand the obvious, that our food and resources come from the earth; but very few of us are connected to the process of planting and harvesting, whether on land or sea. We drain the life out of the earth by siphoning off oil and other natural resources. We rely on fast food windows or glossy store aisles to feed and clothe us.

Consequently, we are not in touch with the natural cycles of the earth for which our bodies are deeply geared. The tides, the seasons, the innate cycles and patterns of the earth are a connection to the very core of our human bodies. So get connected!

This is a very simple exercise. Get outside! Walk, stomp, or run on the earth. Swim in the lakes, oceans, and rivers. Climb trees and mountains, and get some sunshine, your best source of vitamin D. Take a tip from Morticia from the *Addams Family* television show and get a "moon bath." Sit under a carpet of stars, drink in the moon's light, and connect with both the earth upon which you sit and the celestial bodies above you.

Breathing In Nature's Power

When you are out in nature, pounding the earth and loving it, take a few moments and do this simple exercise. You may sit or stand, whichever is more comfortable for you. Look at the ground or water in front of you, or gaze toward a spectacular vista.

Take some deep breaths into your body, drawing the breath down as far as you can within your body. Exhale slowly. Now foster with your mind and intuition a connection to the dynamic life-force energy, or chi, which exists within and animates all things. Connect with all the things in nature that surround you.

Breathe that energy into every pore of your body and exhale back out the same way. Continue this way of breathing for as long as you like, using slow and steady breaths. Don't worry if you cannot focus on the entirety of your body in the beginning. Simply hold a soft focus rather than gluing your attention to a certain section of your body. Just breathe it all in, and exhale any tension, disease, or imbalance from your body. Breathe in freshness, strength, and vitality. This is a form of whole-body breathing. It will vivify every part of you.

Visualizing Optimal Well-Being

Sit in a comfortable position or lie down. Center yourself by taking a few deep breaths. Now visualize your body in its most complete and well state standing in front of you or floating above you, whichever is appropriate to your body's posture.

Once you have that image, light up that body with red, the color of the first chakra. Still visualizing the optimal shape and wellness of your body, intensify the red color and really make it vibrate with life-force energy. When your intuition and body's wisdom tell you to do so, allow that red energy body to slip into your physical body, like a hand slipping into a glove. Fully see, feel, hear, and know the power of a well-balanced physical body, aglow and charged with red first-chakra energy, now inside your physical body.

Repeat this process using all the chakra colors (red, orange, yellow, green, sky blue, indigo, and violet). Follow whatever order is directed by your intuition. If you are guided to do only one or a couple of the chakras, that is perfectly fine. As always, commit to your wisdom and trust what you are given. You can even ask your body if you need to add additional colors to a particular chakra to bring about further wellness and balance.

You might be directed to incorporate this exercise into your daily life, or on the other hand, weekly or even less frequently; however often, it will be appropriate to you and bring the healing your body desires.

Draining Unwanted Energy from Your Body

You probably get tired and worn out at times—we all do. One of the causes of fatigue is holding onto too much energy from other people and situations in your daily life. It is therefore wise to release what is not yours; you will feel lighter and less encumbered.

To drain unwanted energy from your body, sit or stand with your feet hip-width apart. Draw in two or three deep breaths through your nose, dropping the energy and focus of your breath all the way into the pelvic area. Exhale slowly through your mouth. Now, with a steady, focused breath, visualize roots or cords dropping from the soles of your feet into the earth. While staying grounded, breathing gently but deeply, take the focus of your attention to your seventh, or crown, chakra. Ask your body what color or combination of colors you need to run through it to drain away all that is not yours. Listen and trust what you get. Take the color(s) and form a ball of energy slightly above your crown chakra. Then allow the color(s) to flow into the crown chakra, down your arms, and out the palms of your hands. (This is similar to a reverse, modified Running the Rainbow.) Continue with the colored energy running through your torso and down your legs, out the soles of your feet, and through your grounding cords.

Now here is the key: Once you have the energy flowing through your body in this way, know that it will continue as you move to the next step. Take your attention to your heart center. Ask it where any unwanted energy, either yours or someone else's, is located in your body. Listen and follow your heart center's guidance to the location(s) of this unwanted energy. If you find more than one location, take them one at a time; you will be guided as to which locations need to be addressed, which color or colors will be needed, and in what order.

Ask the unwanted energy if it has anything to tell you. Listen and trust. Then, when you are confident that the dialogue with this unwanted energy has run its course, bless it, bless and release anyone or anything that is attached to it, and allow the unwanted energy to flow down the grounding cord or roots extending from your feet and into the earth, thus draining away energy that is not helpful to you.

Repeat this process as many times as you need to until you have worked on all the locations in your body that are storing unwanted energy. You don't need this type of congestion; it only leads to misalignments and disorders, so release it. Again, as you go from location to location, be aware that the colors may change. Your liver area, for example, might need red to run through your body, while your lower back may need a combination of green and blue. Trust your body's wisdom; do as you are guided to most effectively drain away obstructive energy.

The Power of Movement

Whatever calls to you, do it, whether it's yoga (and there are many flavors of yoga today available for sampling), tai chi, qigong, biking, rowing, weight lifting, jogging, dance, or anything. The energy in your personal energy system will circulate as you move your body. Any congestion in the organs and your digestive tract will be able to better cleanse itself for improved health. Your blood will not be so filled with toxins seeping in from an unhealthy small intestinal tract or colon. Honor your body and move it. Don't wait until your body shakes you up by screaming at you through a disorder or disease; instead, ask your body what sort of movement or exercise it would like to engage in—and do it.

While you are out there moving your body, breathe. Breathe deeply, dropping the energy of your breath into your pelvic area. Breathing in this way will help restore and revitalize your body through increased oxygenation. Inhale deeply through the nostrils, feeling, seeing, and knowing that you are dropping the energy of your breath to your body's pelvic floor. Then exhale through the mouth, sending the air out of your body with a quick, strong HAH. Inhaling and releasing the breath through the body in this manner will shift more energy and thought forms.

Here's how it works: When you move your body, you are mainly engaging the consciousness levels of the lower three chakras, since they govern the physical realm. When you bring the breath deep into the body, energetically bouncing your breath off the first chakra, you clear the negative thought forms that are stirred up as you move your body. At the same time, you reinforce the positive ones.

If, for example, you currently weigh a little more than you want or your body is not in its best form, pay attention to the thoughts streaming through your mind when you start moving your body. Are they telling you how out of shape you are, insulting you? Know that as you hear them they are offering you an opportunity to release them. Breathe them away. Breathe down into the first chakra (keep in mind that you have to get through the upper chakras to get there, so it affects them as well) and hold the intention of releasing all negative thoughts that have held you back in the past. In this way, use the power of your breath, your mind, the will of your spirit (which holds your truth), and the movement of your body to release the negativity from it.

When you work on the level of the body to release things, you will also move your life—dramatically. After all, we are in a physical world that needs to be dealt with. If you ignore your physical body, sooner or later it will come to settle accounts. In three-dimensional realty, because it is your soul's mouthpiece, the body commands attention.

Protecting Your Spirit

One of the more common energetic protection techniques is to place a bubble of light—any color of light, but white is used most often—around your physical body. You can make this bubble of light as large or as tight fitting around the physical body as you like. I would also suggest that you have the base of the bubble stretch beneath your feet far enough to really cover you from head to toe, as if it were your cocoon.

While I am teaching and encouraging you to use this technique no matter where you are on your path of evolution, your own spiritual practice will eventually be your natural source of protection. Nonetheless, use the bubble protection technique as a tool in situations where you feel you need it, or if you need a little extra boost to ward off the external stimuli that are constantly pounding your energetic field. It is always good to seek a little more protection if you know you are stepping into a situation where you understand your energy may be compromised.

The bubble is simply a way of describing the shield of protection that you can create by focusing your attention on your electromagnetic field. When you are holding the intention to surround yourself with protective light and energy, you are expanding your field as well as creating a clear boundary around yourself.

Other forms of spiritual protection are also available to you. After I work with diseases that are heavily charged energetically or pervasive in someone's body, I often wash my hands with salt water. Salt is alkaline in nature, and disease is acidic. If you are doing energetic healing work and have contact with disorders related to the immune system and other biochemical imbalances, it is a good idea to wash up with salt water. Sea salt is my first choice; regular table salt, Epsom salts, and baking soda follow.

Whether you do healing work or not, take advantage of the purifying salts of ocean water and take a warm sea salt bath, especially if you have had a particularly rough day. Mix in some herbs or fragrant oils and relax in the healing water. If you are a shower person or don't have enough time to soak in the tub, pour some sea salt into the palm of your hand and rub it over your body. Always pay particular attention to the chakras, front and back, as well as any specific areas your intuitive wisdom guides you to.

You can also wear white sage on your body for protection. Slip it into a shirt pocket, your bra, or your pants pocket. For convenience, you can create little sage sacks. Simply take natural cloth and cut it into four-by-four-inch squares and place a small amount of sage in the center. You can either roll it and tie it with string or sew the edges of the two squares together. You can then place these sage sacks in your dresser drawers to protect your personal items or in strategic places throughout your living space. Corners, closets, and areas in your living space that you feel collect energy are excellent places for these sage packets.

You can also burn sage for protection and to clear the energy fields around your body or in your living space. Fill a seashell or heatproof bowl with the sage and light the herb just enough to start a small flame. Then extinguish the flame and allow the smoke from the sage to fill the air in the room or rooms you wish to clear. Burning sage does a wonderful job of clearing and purifying your energetic system as the smoke is lightly fanned throughout your space.

Try burning a wonderful combination of herbs: sage for clearing, lavender for beauty, cedar tips for blessing, and sweetgrass for protection. Simply combine them, light them, and then let the flame extinguish and the smoke fill your living space. When smoking out negative energies in your living space, make sure that you not only act responsibly around the fire, but also open windows or doors to allow both the air and negative energy to move through and out of the space.

I have had instances when I have been attempting to clear space but did not allow for sufficient movement of air. As a result, doors and windows rattled, slammed, and banged around (and not because of windy weather), which of course scared me to death at first. So always check to be sure that there is a good flow of air and energy in a space before you begin clearing it. Negative energy has to have a place to go when you are bringing in a more love- and God-centered energy; make an exit for it by opening a window or door so the forces you don't want in your space can go out peacefully.

Whenever you are doing any clearing and protection of the energetic space around your body or in your living space, say prayers, blessings, and words of gratitude. Call in your God-force energy, your angels, or other divine forces that please and resonate with you. Create a wonderful space for yourself energetically. You'll notice the difference.

Understanding Your Body's Point of View

This is a very simple process, and one that will bring you insights regarding how your body is doing. Sit or lie down. Take a few breaths into your body and relax. With each exhale, let go of the tension in your muscles. Let yourself sink into the chair, floor, couch, or bed.

Intuitively ask which part of your body you need to have a conversation with. If you are currently suffering from an illness, go to that particular region of your body. Also ask if any other part of your body has something to say about this situation. Ask for the highest level of consciousness to speak with you. It is important to hear the more shadowed side of your body's opinion, even though it may be spouting negative talk and criticism rather than helpful healing advice; we need to listen to the disgruntled part of ourselves too. It's like good customer service. You pay attention to the complaints as well as the praise.

This process is about asking questions. Ask simple ones and start your questions with "what" words. *What is going on? What do I need to do to bring about healing? What do you have to tell me?*

Just have a conversation with your body. It will tell you what you need to know. Your task is to listen, trust, and follow through with any actions that are necessary for your healing. It's also valuable to jot down the answers you get. Sometimes when you do this, you'll end up in a relaxed state of mind, which is great; but you may not remember all that you discovered. If you like, use a tape recorder. Just press Record and set it on your chest or lap. Vocalize your questions and speak out loud the answers you hear.

Clearing Energetic Impacts

I have found through experience that this is a powerful exercise. It came to me during a time when I was healing the lingering effects of a broken right ankle. It had healed reasonably well, but I had lost a great deal of flexibility in it and in my foot. Since I do yoga as a part of my personal practice and teach it in the context of workshops, I was a bit discouraged by this loss. I went to a traditional medical doctor. After viewing a $1,200 MRI, he concluded that I had lost movement in my foot and the only recourse was to perform surgery, which might or might not work. My inner physician, however, told me there was another way, that I could engage energy medicine to fix the problem. I left the doctor's office and went home.

The next afternoon, I lay on my healing table and told God to give me some direction. I'm still a little bossy sometimes with the universal forces. Nonetheless, my request was granted. This chakra breath exercise was the result of that request.

I followed the instructions I had received through my meditation, which I repeat below. First, however, I'll describe my initial experience with this exercise, the process, and its results. I took three breaths of pink energy into my mouth and visualized them dropping down my spinal column and into the second chakra region. I held each breath for a moment or two, while holding the intention for complete healing. (Note: Second-chakra energy/consciousness is also manifested in the wrists and ankles.) I exhaled my pink, energized breath out the back of my second chakra, doing as my body directed. While I was exhaling the third breath, much to my surprise, my right ankle snapped into alignment. Ever since that moment, I have enjoyed full movement of my right foot and ankle, with no pain or stiffness. Needless to say, I was amazed and grateful. I also ran to my computer to copy down the instructions for this exercise so I could share it with my clients and now with you.

When I am working with an individual on correcting rifts in his or her chakras, I use this exercise most often. As you will see, it is not limited to working with one particular chakra or part of the body. While attending a client in person, I usually suggest the order in which to work with each chakra. Since I am not personally with you, however, you will have to be your own healing facilitator. And because you already are that, simply ask your body in which order you should work with your chakras. Just ask, listen, and trust. The ideal order will be revealed to you. Before proceeding, jot down in your journal the order your body gave you regarding working with your chakras.

Once you have the order established, you will need to create the setup for working with each chakra. The setup is as follows:

1. If your body has guided you to work with a particular chakra, ask whether you need to work with the front or the back of it. (This applies only to chakras two through six, since they have both a front and a back.) You can also ask your body if you need to work with a particular organ such as your stomach, heart, or liver.

2. Ask what color or combination of colors you need to incorporate into your breath for the purpose of the exercise. More than likely, the colors will change each time you do this exercise. This is because different colors have different vibrational rates applicable to the variety of subtle levels of healing required for specific conditions; a color or combination of colors will mix with your breath (*prana*, or life-force energy) and provide healing to a specific chakra.

3. Ask how many breaths of colored energy you need for this particular session. (As with the colors, the number of breaths will likely change each time you do this exercise.) Also ask if you need to exhale the breath out the front or back of the body; you could also hold the color in, as you exhale naturally. When your body instructs you to do this, visualize the colors(s) being packed into the organ or chakra.

Note: Do not strain yourself while holding your breath. If you become dizzy, do not do this exercise. Once you have ascertained the above information, you are ready to proceed as follows.

Visualize the colors you have been told to use floating in a cloud in front of your face. Gently inhale, drawing the colored energy into the back of your throat, sipping the energy into your body. Now, while gently holding your breath, visualize that ball of colored energy dropping down your spinal column to the specific chakra location, or organ, with which you are working. Continue to hold your breath and the intention of experiencing release and blessing. As you are exhaling, see, feel, hear, or know the energy and breath as they move from the spine into the narrow opening of the chakra where it attaches to the spine and then out through the body of that chakra. Repeat as needed. (Since the spine ends below the head, when you work on the sixth and seventh chakras, simply breathe into your entire head, filling it with colored energy. As you exhale, focus the colored energy in the center of the brain and release it out the appropriate chakra.)

Because this exercise can clear the energetic impact that caused a rift in your chakra system—an event you might not even recollect—you may not have a lot of cognitive processing to do during or after, and that is the special magic of this exercise. If something comes up that you feel you need to deal with, however, either by yourself or with a trained therapist, do so; as I've said many times, follow your body's wisdom and be well.

"What Do I Do Now?"

A special invitation to accelerate your intuition

I have shared principles and tools in the fields of intuitive development and energy medicine. With practice, you will awaken the ability to sense life from a fabulous perspective. When you take charge of your intuition and your energy, you throw open the doors of change in the areas of relationships, finances, health, and career. You are naturally intuitive! You can heal yourself and change your reality.

As with any subject matter, intuition needs to be experienced and guided before its wisdom can generate a deep transformation. Yes, you can do this on your own; and I encourage you to do so. Nonetheless, group work truly accelerates learning, and there is instant feedback as you practice with others in intuitively-driven processes. It is a profound experience!

As a facilitator, I want you to succeed, to be the best you can be, and to achieve your dreams. Therefore, I wish to extend my commitment to you beyond this book by offering the opportunity to take action and to elevate your intuitive skills to a new and astounding level. Simply go to www.energymedicine.org and click on the "Featured Seminar" link. There you will find a special gift that will make accelerating your intuition and healing skills more attainable.

I sincerely thank you for your commitment to yourself and to your learning. It takes courage to step toward a new horizon. I commend you for your passion to accomplish this and to allow your intuitive power to flower and flourish. You will help not only yourself, but others as well. That is the ultimate goal—to be of service.

All best wishes to you and yours,
Laura Alden Kamm